Your Fertility Blueprint is the empowering, science-backed guide every woman deserves on her fertility journey. Dr. Stephanie Gray beautifully bridges her personal experience with evidence-based functional medicine, giving hope to women who've been dismissed or told "everything looks normal." I love how she shines a light on the critical gut–uterus connection—a concept too often overlooked in conventional medicine—and gives practical, compassionate steps to help women uncover and heal the root causes of infertility. This book is a must-read for anyone who wants to understand her body more deeply, advocate for herself, and reclaim her reproductive health.

—Dr. Tabatha Barber, DO, FACOOG, NCMP, IFMCP
Best-Selling Author, Founder and CEO of Fast to Faith®

Your Fertility Blueprint is the playbook I wish every couple had on day one-clear, compassionate, and fiercely practical. Dr. Stephanie Gray turns overwhelm into action with a step-by-step, functional medicine plan that actually gets to root causes and restores hope. If you're ready to stop guessing and start building your healthiest path to a family, this is your blueprint.

— JJ Virgin, CNS, BCHN, EP-C, New York Times Bestselling Author of *The Virgin Diet* and *JJ Virgin's Sugar Impact Diet*

Dr. Stephanie Gray's *Your Fertility Blueprint* is a game-changer for anyone navigating the complexities of fertility. As a Holistic Fertility Specialist for close to 15 years, I'm continually searching for resources that bridge evidence-based medicine with a truly integrative and holistic approach.

Stephanie's personal journey and integrative protocols empower readers and practitioners alike to ask the right questions and look beyond conventional care—especially for those facing unexplained infertility or recurrent pregnancy loss. Her deep dive into functional medicine testing and underlying root causes makes this book an invaluable resource on the journey to optimal reproductive health. I highly recommend *Your Fertility Blueprint* to anyone seeking answers, hope, and a clear action plan for optimizing their fertility and overall well-being.

— **Dr. Aumatma Simmons, Holistic Fertility Specialist, TEDx Speaker, "Egg Meets Sperm" Podcast Host, Author of** *Fertility Secrets: What Your Doctor Didn't Tell You About Babymaking*

As a physician studying the impact of past trauma on our body and biology, I recognize the profound truth that Dr. Gray has contained within these pages. This blueprint provides the biological roadmap that many other fertility approaches miss. This book is essential reading for anyone whose body has been saying 'not yet' to new life.

— **Dr. Aimie Apigian, MD, MS, MPH National Bestselling Author of** *The Biology of Trauma,* **Leading Expert in Trauma, Attachment, and the Nervous System**

Dr. Gray has created an invaluable resource that bridges the gap between conventional fertility treatments and functional medicine. This book provides both patients and practitioners with practical, evidence-based strategies that can transform fertility outcomes. This a must-read for anyone working in reproductive health.

—Tracy Gapin, MD, FACS, Founder and CEO of Peak Launch & Gapin Institute for Precision Medicine

Dr. Gray has written a book that makes a confusing and stressful topic feel clear and hopeful. *Your Fertility Blueprint* gives readers easy-to-follow steps, real science, and a caring voice. It's a guide that helps both patients and providers see a new way forward with fertility—practical, thoughtful, and full of heart.

—Deb Matthew, MD, America's Happy Hormones Doctor

Your Fertility Blueprint is a must-read for anyone navigating the often-overwhelming world of fertility challenges. This book is a beautiful blend of evidence-based functional medicine protocols and a deeply personal journey of persistence and advocacy. It offers a comprehensive roadmap for uncovering the root causes of unexplained infertility and recurrent pregnancy loss, addressing everything from underlying infections and inflammatory conditions to blood clotting disorders and beyond.

As someone who has walked alongside countless women on their fertility journeys, I deeply appreciate the actionable insights and compassionate guidance this book provides. It empowers both patients and practitioners to think beyond standard fertility evaluations and embrace a more integrative, holistic approach to reproductive health. This is more than a book—it's a lifeline for those seeking answers and hope. I highly recommend it!

— **Anna Cabeca, DO, OBGYN, FACOG, bestselling author of** *The Hormone Fix*

From the moment I met Dr. Stephanie Gray, I knew I had found my expert for women's health, hormones, and fertility. Her knowledge stems from years of clinical experience, extensive study, and her personal journey. For complex hormonal cases, Dr. Gray always provided the solution. Her first book, *Your Longevity Blueprint*, is my go-to guide for patients seeking to optimize their health and longevity. Now, *Your Fertility Blueprint* offers a masterful integration of functional medicine principles to optimize both fertility and overall health. Dr. Gray is a brilliant clinician with a passionate heart for human health and flourishing. I strongly recommend this book for patients and practitioners seeking to understand the complex variables influencing human fertility.

— **David A. Vickery, MD, Authentic Health**

YOUR FERTILITY
BLUEPRINT

YOUR FERTILITY BLUEPRINT

RENOVATING YOUR REPRODUCTIVE HEALTH
THROUGH **FUNCTIONAL MEDICINE**

DR. STEPHANIE GRAY

Copyright ©2025 Dr. Stephanie Gray.
All rights reserved.

No part of this publication may be reproduced or transmitted in any form or by any means, electronic or mechanical, including photography, recording, or any information storage and retrieval system, without permission in writing from the author. Requests for permission to make copies of any part of the work should be emailed to the following address: info@ihhclinic.com.

Neither the publisher nor the author shall be liable for any loss of profit or any other commercial damages, including but not limited to special, incidental, consequential, personal, or other damages.

Published and distributed by Blueprint Health & Family Press
Marion, USA

Library of Congress Control Number: 2025913570
Gray, Stephanie
Your Fertility Blueprint: Renovating Your Reproductive Health through Functional Medicine

ISBN
Paperback 979-8-9993023-0-4
eBook 979-8-9993023-1-1

Graphic design by Jessie Counts

To William and Michael, my two precious miracles—you were worth every prayer, every tear, and every moment of the ten-year journey that brought you into our lives. This book exists because of you and for you.

To Eric, my partner in faith, love, and life—thank you for never letting me give up on the dream God placed in our hearts. Your unwavering belief sustained me when mine faltered.

And to every woman and man who has ever felt the ache of an empty womb, the disappointment of another negative test, or the fear that their dream might never come true—this blueprint is for you.
Your miracle is waiting.

"He gives the childless woman a family, making her a happy mother."
— Psalm 113:9

MEDICAL DISCLAIMER AND AUTHOR'S QUALIFICATIONS

The information contained in this book is based on my experience as an Advanced Registered Nurse Practitioner (ARNP) since 2009, with a doctorate in nursing focusing on estrogen metabolism (2011), masters in Metabolic Nutritional Medicine (2013) and fellowship training in anti-aging, regenerative, and functional medicine (completed in 2013), combined with over sixteen years of clinical practice and my personal fertility journey.

I am not an obstetrician-gynecologist or reproductive endocrinologist. The content in this book represents functional and integrative medicine approaches to fertility optimization and should not replace conventional medical care when appropriate. During my own fertility journey, I worked with both OB-GYNs and reproductive endocrinologists while simultaneously applying functional medicine principles—an integrative approach that ultimately led to my success.

This book is intended for educational purposes and to share evidence-based functional medicine strategies that can complement conventional fertility care. Always consult with qualified healthcare providers, including reproductive specialists when indicated, before implementing any new protocols or making significant changes to your health regimen.

Identifying details for patient case studies I shared have been changed to protect privacy.

FOREWORD

This book exists because of grace, love, and the unwavering support of people who believed in our dream when we could barely hold onto it ourselves.

First and foremost, I thank God for the knowledge, wisdom, and calling He has placed on my life to serve my patients and help families grow. Every insight in these pages, every breakthrough in understanding, every moment of clarity that led to healing—all of it flows from His infinite wisdom. I am simply a vessel, honored to be used in His plan to bring hope and health to those who desperately need it.

To my parents and their incredible network of prayer warriors who faithfully lifted Eric and me up through every month, every disappointment, every procedure, and every glimmer of hope during our decade-long fertility journey—your prayers sustained us when our own faith wavered. You believed for us when we couldn't believe for ourselves. You held our dream in your hearts and carried it to the throne of grace again and again. I know beyond any doubt that your intercession played a vital role in bringing William and Michael into our lives.

To my husband Eric, my partner in every sense of the word—you stood by my side through ten years of fertility struggles with a strength and faith that humbled me daily. While I was consumed with treatments and protocols, you managed our business, supported our patients, and held our family together. When I wanted to give up, you reminded me that God had children for us. When I felt broken, you saw me as whole. This journey tested us in ways we never imagined, but it also showed me what true partnership looks like. I couldn't have walked this path with anyone else.

To my incredible team at the Integrative Health and Hormone Clinic—you are the heartbeat of everything we do. During the countless appointments, procedures, and recovery periods when I needed to step away, you kept our mission alive. You cared for our patients with the same dedication and compassion I would have given them myself. You believed in our functional medicine approach even when others questioned it, and you celebrated every patient success as if it were your own. This work isn't possible without each of you.

But ultimately, I wrote this book for my two miracle sons, William and Michael. One day, when you're old enough to understand, I want you to know the journey that brought you here—not because it was easy, but because it was worth every moment of struggle. I want you to know that you were prayed for, hoped for, and fought for long before you drew your first breath. And I want you to understand that sometimes the most precious gifts come wrapped in the longest waits.

I also wrote this book for every couple who is walking the path Eric and I walked—feeling alone, confused, and wondering if their dreams will ever become reality. I wrote it for the woman lying awake at 3 a.m., googling unexplained infertility for the hundredth time. I wrote it for the man watching his wife's heart break month after month, feeling helpless to fix it. I wrote it for the couples sitting in fertility clinic waiting rooms, wondering if there's another way.

My deepest prayer is that this book will shorten your journey, that the knowledge that took me years to piece together will be available to you from day one, and that you won't have to spend a decade searching for answers that could be found in months with the right approach.

If this blueprint helps even one couple avoid the pain of unexplained infertility, if it guides even one person to discover their missing piece of the fertility puzzle, if it offers even one family hope when they're ready to give up—then every moment of our struggle will have served a purpose greater than ourselves.

May God bless your journey, strengthen your faith, and fulfill the desires of your heart.

With endless gratitude and hope,
Dr. Stephanie Gray

CONTENTS

FOREWORD	I

SECTION I: INTRODUCTION: BREAKING GROUND ON YOUR FERTILITY FOUNDATION — 1
1. Foundation Planning — 3
2. Understanding the Crisis — 9
3. Blueprint Development and Implementation — 19

SECTION II: STRUCTURAL INTEGRITY—THE HOLISTIC IMPACT OF HORMONE BALANCE ON FERTILITY — 31
4. The Foundation Systems—Biological and Psychological Aspects of Fertility — 33
5. The Social Architecture—Family Dynamics and Cultural Context in Fertility — 45
6. Creating Sacred Space—Spiritual Dimensions of the Fertility Journey — 55

SECTION III: ENGINEERING THE SYSTEMS—UNDERSTANDING REPRODUCTIVE HORMONES — 67
7. System Architecture—Anatomy and Climate Control — 69
8. Primary Power Systems — 81
9. Support and Environmental Systems — 89
10. System Integration—Monthly Patterns and Assessment — 99

SECTION IV: STRUCTURAL CHALLENGES—DIAGNOSING AND ADDRESSING FERTILITY OBSTACLES — 111
11. Common Structural Issues — 113
12. System Failures and Transitions — 143
13. Hidden Structural Problems and Circulation Issues — 173
14. Integration Challenges—Comprehensive Infertility Assessment — 225
15. Medical Construction Methods — 239
16. Advanced Medical Interventions — 241

SECTION V: DIY FERTILITY IMPROVEMENTS—OPTIMIZING YOUR REPRODUCTIVE HOME — 253
    17 Structural Foundation Work — 255
    18 Quality Materials—Nutrition and Egg Quality Enhancement — 271
    19 Complete Environmental and Nutritional Optimization — 295
    20 Body Work and Energy Systems — 307
    21 Implementation and Professional Support — 321

SECTION VI: CONCLUSION—THE COMPLETED PROJECT — 333
    22 Success Stories and Future Planning — 335

APPENDIX — 349

DOWNLOADABLE RESOURCES — 357

ACKNOWLEDGMENTS — 359

REFERENCES — 363

INDEX — 381

ABOUT THE AUTHOR — 391

SECTION I: INTRODUCTION

BREAKING GROUND ON YOUR FERTILITY FOUNDATION

CHAPTER 1

FOUNDATION PLANNING

THE FOUNDATION OF YOUR FERTILITY JOURNEY

Sarah sat across from me, tears welling in her eyes as she recounted her third miscarriage. At 34, she had been trying to conceive for over two years. "Everyone keeps telling me to just relax and it will happen," she said, frustration evident in her voice. "But I know something's wrong. I can feel it. And no one seems to be listening."

Like Sarah, Emma had also experienced repeated pregnancy losses. At 38, she'd had two miscarriages within a year and was desperate for answers. Her conventional fertility workups showed "nothing wrong," yet she couldn't maintain a pregnancy beyond eight weeks.

Then there was Jennifer, who at 42 had been told by three different reproductive specialists that her only path to motherhood was through donor eggs. Her FSH levels were elevated, her AMH was barely detectable, and according to conventional wisdom, her chances of conceiving with her own eggs were less than 5%.

These stories might sound familiar to you. Perhaps you're experiencing your own fertility challenges—the monthly disappointment, the well-meaning but unhelpful advice from friends and family, the growing anxiety as time passes, and the medical system that seems more focused on technological interventions than finding the root cause of your fertility obstacles.

What connects Sarah, Emma, and Jennifer—besides their struggle to conceive—is that they all eventually found their way to functional medicine. And all three went on to have healthy pregnancies and babies, even Jennifer at age 43, despite being told her own eggs were no longer viable.

How? By addressing the underlying imbalances in their bodies that were preventing conception or causing pregnancy loss. By treating their reproductive systems not as isolated entities but as integrated parts of a whole body ecosystem. By recognizing that fertility isn't just about having functioning reproductive organs but about *creating an internal environment where life can flourish.*

This is the essence of the functional medicine approach to fertility—and it's the foundation of this book.

THE MASTER BLUEPRINT: EXPANDING YOUR LONGEVITY BLUEPRINT FOUNDATION

If you've read my first book, *Your Longevity Blueprint,* you're already familiar with the house metaphor I use to explain how the various systems in your body work together to create health. Just as a well-built home requires proper foundations, structural integrity, electrical wiring, heating and cooling, clog-free plumbing, and a strong roof, your body needs properly functioning digestive, nervous, detoxification, hormonal, cardiovascular, and immune systems to achieve optimal health and longevity.

In *Your Longevity Blueprint*, I introduced the concept that your endocrine system—the network of glands that produce hormones—functions like your body's heating and cooling system. When this system isn't working properly—when your hormones are imbalanced—you simply don't feel well. Just as a malfunctioning HVAC system might leave some rooms in your house too hot while others remain freezing, hormonal imbalances can create a host of seemingly unrelated symptoms throughout your body.

In this book, *Your Fertility Blueprint*, we're going to take that heating and cooling metaphor and expand it, focusing specifically on the impact of hormonal balance on reproductive function. We'll explore how your body's climate control system directly influences your ability to conceive and maintain a healthy pregnancy.

Think of this book as a specialized addition to your master blueprint—a detailed section focusing exclusively on the renovation and optimization of your reproductive systems. While *Your Longevity Blueprint* provided the overall architectural plans for your health, *Your Fertility Blueprint* offers specialized plans for creating and nurturing new life. Your Functional medicine provider will serve as your fertility renovation specialist or contractor, and just as no contractor would begin building without first examining the existing structure, we'll start by assessing your current fertility foundation—identifying strengths to build upon and weaknesses that need addressing before construction can begin.

SITE ASSESSMENT: MY PERSONAL FERTILITY CHALLENGES

Before I guide you through your fertility renovation, I want to share my own renovation story—because I, too, have faced the challenges of creating a solid fertility foundation.

My journey to motherhood wasn't the straightforward path I had envisioned. Despite helping countless patients overcome their fertility obstacles, I found myself facing my own reproductive challenges. After years of hormonal imbalances that I worked to correct through functional medicine approaches, I still encountered obstacles when trying to conceive. I had already tried hCG and progesterone, yet I was still at a fertility standstill.

The irony wasn't lost on me—the provider who specialized in helping others achieve pregnancy was struggling with her own fertility. Like many of my patients, I experienced the emotional roller coaster, the questioning, and the determination to find answers. And like them, I had to apply the principles of functional medicine to my own body.

My personal fertility blueprint required addressing several key issues:

First, I discovered through testing that my body was reacting to gluten and dairy, creating underlying inflammation that affected my reproductive system. Eliminating these foods was my first step toward creating a more hospitable environment for conception.

Next, my testing revealed that years of environmental exposures had led to an accumulation of toxins in my system that can interfere with hormone function. Little did I know that all those chemical hair straighteners, Bath and Body Works products, aluminum-laced deodorant, and chlorine-laced tampons I had been using had all worked against my ability to conceive one day. A change to clean personal care products and a structured detoxification protocol, including infrared sauna sessions and targeted supplements, helped clear these obstacles.

Additionally, like many women in demanding professions, I had to address the chronic stress that was disrupting my hormonal harmony. Incorporating yoga, mindfulness practices, and boundary-setting into my life wasn't just self-care—it was an essential component of my fertility plan.

I also pursued two laparoscopic surgeries and tried several intrauterine inseminations (IUIs).

Moving from what I will never know for sure but what I suspect was a moldy office to a new office was the final hurdle in conceiving William, my first son.

Finally, to bring Michael, my second son, into this world, as you will hear, I did explore more conventional fertility treatments that initially were all unsuccessful until I worked on my uterine mobility, discovered I needed blood thinners, and treated a chronic uterine infection.

I spent a decade on my fertility journey and became so very wary at times (like I'm sure you have) that I nearly gave up.

I share this personal story not to focus on myself, but to emphasize that I understand both professionally and personally the challenges you may be facing. The strategies in this book aren't just theoretical concepts I've studied or approaches I've used with patients—they're the same principles I've applied in my own life to overcome fertility obstacles.

My journey reminds me daily that fertility challenges don't discriminate based on medical knowledge or professional expertise. They affect women and men from all walks of life, and they almost always have physiological roots that can be addressed with the right approach. And I'm not alone. As you will read below, infertility rates are skyrocketing.

CHAPTER 2

UNDERSTANDING THE CRISIS

THE GROWING FERTILITY CRISIS: WHY THIS BOOK MATTERS

Before we begin our journey through your fertility blueprint, it's essential to understand the scope of the fertility challenges facing our society today. What you may be experiencing is not an isolated struggle—you are part of a growing demographic facing unprecedented reproductive challenges.

THE RISING TIDE OF INFERTILITY

The statistics paint a sobering picture:
- **1 in 6 couples worldwide** now struggle with infertility—defined as the inability to conceive after one year of trying—according to the World Health Organization.
- **Female infertility has increased by 25%** since the early 2000s, while **male fertility has declined by over 50% in the past 40 years**, with sperm counts dropping dramatically across Western nations.

- **Secondary infertility**—the inability to conceive after having one or more children—now accounts for approximately 50% of infertility cases, demonstrating that even those who have conceived before are not immune to this growing crisis.
- **Miscarriage rates have risen to affect 15-20%** of known pregnancies, with recurrent pregnancy loss becoming increasingly common.
- **The average age of first conception has risen to 30+** in many developed countries, adding age-related fertility challenges to the equation.
- **IVF success rates remain at approximately 25-30%** per cycle for women under 35, and drop significantly with age—yet more people than ever require assisted reproductive technologies.

These aren't just numbers—they represent millions of individuals and couples experiencing profound grief, frustration, and often financial strain in their quest to create families. The question we must ask is: **Why?** Why are we seeing such dramatic changes in human fertility in just a few generations?

THE PERFECT STORM: WHY FERTILITY IS DECLINING

The answer lies in a convergence of factors creating a perfect storm for reproductive health:

Environmental Factors:
- Unprecedented exposure to endocrine-disrupting chemicals in our food, water, and everyday products
- Microplastics now detected in human blood, placenta, and reproductive tissues

- Heavy metal accumulation, affecting hormonal signaling and egg/sperm quality
- Electromagnetic field exposure from ubiquitous technology

Lifestyle Changes:
- Chronic stress levels at historic highs, directly impacting reproductive hormone production
- Sleep disruption and circadian rhythm dysfunction affecting fertility hormones
- Increasingly sedentary lifestyles altering metabolism and hormonal balance
- Delayed childbearing as more couples prioritize career and financial stability first

Nutritional Shifts:
- Processed food diets lacking the key nutrients needed for reproduction
- Soil depletion resulting in foods with fewer minerals and vitamins
- Gut microbiome disruption from antibiotics, food additives, and stress
- Inflammatory dietary patterns compromising reproductive tissue function

Medical Factors:
- Rising rates of undiagnosed thyroid disorders directly impacting fertility
- Increased prevalence of autoimmune conditions affecting reproductive function

- More women experiencing hormone-related conditions like Polycystic Ovary Syndrome (PCOS) and endometriosis
- Growing evidence of intergenerational effects—your parents' exposures affecting your fertility

Conventional Healthcare Limitations:
- Focus on symptom management rather than addressing root causes
- Tendency to normalize reproductive symptoms like painful periods and PMS
- Limited testing that misses subclinical hormone imbalances
- Few options between "keep trying" and expensive assisted reproductive technologies

This complex interplay of factors explains why even health-conscious individuals—people who exercise, maintain healthy weights, and eat reasonably well—often struggle with fertility. Our reproductive systems simply weren't designed to handle this unprecedented combination of challenges.

In this increasingly challenging reproductive landscape, the **conventional** medical approach—while valuable for many—often **falls short** for several reasons:

1. **It treats symptoms rather than systems**—addressing individual hormone imbalances without examining why they occurred
2. **It compartmentalizes the body**—separating reproductive health from digestive, immune, and neurological function

3. **It relies primarily on pharmaceutical and technological interventions**—often bypassing the body's natural capacity for healing
4. **It applies standardized protocols**—rather than personalized approaches based on individual biochemistry and circumstances

WHY FUNCTIONAL MEDICINE OFFERS HOPE

Instead, the **functional** medicine approach outlined in this book offers such powerful **hope**. Rather than fighting against your body's natural functions or bypassing them entirely, functional medicine works to restore optimal function to all the interconnected systems that support reproduction.

By addressing the root causes of fertility challenges—inflammation, nutrient depletion, toxin accumulation, stress physiology, hormonal communication, and more—we can often restore natural fertility or significantly improve outcomes with assisted reproductive technologies.

THE POWER OF INTEGRATIVE MEDICINE IN FERTILITY CARE

While functional medicine provides the foundation for addressing root causes of fertility challenges, I believe integrative medicine offers the most comprehensive path forward for many couples. Integrative medicine thoughtfully combines the best of conventional medical treatments with evidence-based complementary and alternative approaches, creating a personalized treatment strategy that honors both scientific rigor and the body's innate healing wisdom. As my personal story illustrates, I successfully utilized both conventional interventions—including laparoscopic surgeries, IUIs, IVF, antibiotics, and blood thinners—alongside functional medicine protocols focused on addressing nutrient deficiencies, inflammation, stress reduction, toxin exposure, and hormonal imbalances. This integrative approach recognizes that while functional medicine excels at identifying and treating the underlying causes of infertility, some women may also benefit from conventional fertility treatments to achieve pregnancy. Rather than viewing these approaches as competing philosophies, **integrative** medicine sees them as complementary tools in a comprehensive fertility toolkit.

By combining conventional medicine's technological advances with functional medicine's root-cause focus and other evidence-based therapies, we can create the most fertile environment possible while utilizing all available resources to help you achieve your dream of parenthood.

A NOTE ON THIS BOOK'S FORMAT

I received excellent feedback for my first book, *Your Longevity Blueprint*, but many readers told me it was a lot to digest. I hated leaving anything out, so I included everything I thought could be helpful—which sometimes made it overwhelming to know where to start or what to prioritize. Learning from that experience, I've intentionally kept this book's format easier to read and apply. You'll notice I use bullet points throughout to break down complex concepts into actionable steps, making it simpler to implement the strategies that will support your fertility journey. My goal is to give you comprehensive information without overwhelming you, so you can focus your energy on healing rather than trying to decode dense medical text.

THIS BOOK'S UNIQUE APPROACH

In the pages that follow, you'll discover a comprehensive approach that:

- **Addresses the entire body**—not just the reproductive organs
- **Considers your unique biochemistry**—not one-size-fits-all protocols
- **Empowers you with practical steps**—not just theoretical knowledge
- **Combines ancient wisdom with cutting-edge science**—not limited to a single paradigm
- **Works with conventional treatments when needed**—embracing an integrative approach rather than an either/or proposition

You'll learn how to systematically "renovate" your reproductive home, creating the optimal environment for conception and healthy pregnancy. And importantly, you'll be improving your overall health in the process—*because true fertility is simply an expression of whole-body wellness.*

Whether you've just started thinking about conception, have been trying for years, or are somewhere in between, this approach offers a path forward that honors your body's innate wisdom while providing practical, evidence-based strategies for overcoming today's unprecedented fertility challenges.

In a world where reproductive health faces more threats than ever before, this functional medicine blueprint provides the comprehensive approach needed to navigate the journey to parenthood. Let's begin.

ARCHITECTURAL PHILOSOPHY: DEFINING FUNCTIONAL MEDICINE FOR REPRODUCTIVE WELLNESS

Before we break ground on your fertility renovation, it's important to understand the architectural philosophy that guides our approach. In *Your Longevity Blueprint*, I compared conventional medicine to the fire department—excellent for putting out fires (acute conditions) with their axes and hoses (drugs and surgery)—but not equipped to rebuild the house afterward or prevent future fires.

This comparison is particularly apt when it comes to reproductive medicine. Conventional fertility treatment often focuses on manipulating or bypassing the reproductive system's natural functions rather than identifying and addressing why those functions aren't working correctly in the first place.

Consider the contrast between approaches:

The Conventional Approach to Fertility:
- Identifies structural problems (blocked tubes, fibroids, etc.)
- Measures hormone levels at specific points
- Classifies patients based on diagnostic categories (PCOS, endometriosis, unexplained infertility)
- Primarily offers treatments that either stimulate or bypass natural function (medication, IUI, IVF)
- Often treats all patients with similar diagnoses using standardized protocols
- Focuses mainly on the reproductive system in isolation

The Functional Medicine Approach to Fertility:
- Examines why structural problems or hormonal imbalances developed
- Assesses hormone patterns, genetics, metabolism, and cellular function
- Views diagnoses as descriptions of symptoms, not root causes
- Offers treatments that restore optimal function to the body's natural systems
- Customizes treatment based on each person's unique biochemistry and circumstances
- Recognizes the reproductive system as integrated with all other body systems

This doesn't mean conventional reproductive treatments don't have their place—they certainly do, and they've helped millions of people build families. Rather, functional medicine offers a complementary approach that can either help you conceive naturally or enhance the effectiveness of conventional treatments by addressing the underlying factors affecting your fertility.

Think of it this way: If your reproductive system is a home in need of renovation, *conventional medicine* fertility treatment might install a powerful new furnace without checking why the old one failed or whether the electrical system can support it. *Functional medicine* examines the entire structure—foundation, wiring, insulation, air quality—to create an environment where the heating system can function optimally on its own, or where the new furnace will have everything it needs to operate efficiently.

In the chapters that follow, we'll explore this integrative approach in detail, examining how each system in your body contributes to reproductive health and how optimizing these systems can enhance your fertility. Just as each component of a house must work in harmony for the structure to be sound, each system in your body must function optimally for fertility to flourish.

CHAPTER 3

BLUEPRINT DEVELOPMENT AND IMPLEMENTATION

THE CLIMATE CONTROL SYSTEM: EXPANDING OUR HEATING AND COOLING METAPHOR

As I mentioned earlier, in *Your Longevity Blueprint*, I compared your endocrine system to your home's heating and cooling system. When functioning properly, this climate control system maintains comfortable temperatures throughout your house. Similarly, your endocrine system regulates everything from metabolism to mood, energy to sleep, and of course, reproduction.

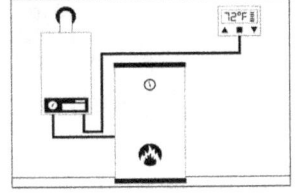

For fertility purposes, we need to expand this metaphor to understand the specific ways your hormonal climate control system affects your ability to conceive and maintain pregnancy.

Imagine your reproductive system as a greenhouse within your home—a specialized environment where new life can take root and flourish.

This greenhouse requires even more precise climate control than the rest of the house. The temperature must be exact, humidity levels carefully maintained, and air quality pristine for seeds to germinate and plants to thrive.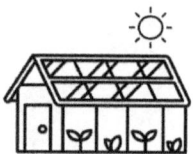

Your reproductive hormones function as this specialized climate control system. Estrogen, progesterone, testosterone, follicle stimulating hormone (FSH), luteinizing hormone (LH), thyroid hormones, cortisol, insulin, and others work in a delicate balance to create the perfect conditions for conception. When this system functions optimally:

- Follicles develop properly (seeds mature)
- Ovulation occurs regularly (seeds are ready for pollination)
- The uterine lining develops with adequate thickness and blood supply (soil is nutrient-rich)
- Cervical mucus becomes hospitable to sperm (the path to pollination is clear)
- After conception, hormone levels adjust to maintain pregnancy (the greenhouse environment adapts to nurture the sprouting seed)

However, just as a greenhouse's climate control can malfunction in various ways, your reproductive hormone system can develop different types of imbalances, several of which I struggled with:

- **Too cold in some areas:** Low estrogen or thyroid function can lead to inadequate follicular development or thin uterine lining
- **Too hot in others:** Excess androgens in conditions like PCOS can prevent proper ovulation
- **Irregular temperature fluctuations:** Erratic hormone levels can lead to unpredictable cycles
- **Poor humidity control:** Imbalances affecting cervical mucus production can create barriers to conception
- **Inadequate air circulation:** Issues with blood flow to reproductive organs can affect egg quality and implantation
- **Control system malfunctions:** Problems with the hypothalamic-pituitary axis can disrupt the signals controlling the entire system

Throughout this book, we'll examine these various "climate control malfunctions" in detail, explaining how they affect your fertility and—most importantly—how to repair them to create the optimal environment for conception.

BUILDING YOUR PERSONAL FERTILITY BLUEPRINT

Now that we understand the architectural philosophy guiding our approach and have expanded our heating and cooling metaphor specifically for fertility, let's discuss how to develop your personal fertility blueprint.

Just as an architect doesn't create the same house design for every client, there's no one-size-fits-all plan for optimizing fertility. **Let me repeat that again. There is no one-size-fits-all plan for optimizing fertility regardless of what you've been told.** Your blueprint must be customized based on your unique body, health history, and specific fertility challenges.

The development of your personal fertility blueprint begins with a thorough assessment:

1. COMPREHENSIVE TESTING

In my clinic, I use a range of functional medicine tests to identify the underlying factors affecting fertility. These may include:

- **Detailed Hormone Panels:** Beyond the standard day-3 FSH and LH, we examine hormone patterns throughout the cycle, including estrogens, progesterone, androgens, and their metabolites
- **Thyroid Function:** Comprehensive thyroid panels including free T3, free T4, reverse T3, and thyroid antibodies
- **Adrenal Function:** Cortisol patterns throughout the day and DHEA levels
- **Nutritional Status:** Testing for vitamins, minerals, antioxidants, fatty acids, and amino acids critical for reproductive function
- **Digestive Function:** Assessing gut health, which influences hormone metabolism and immune function
- **Toxin Burden:** Evaluating environmental toxin exposure that may disrupt hormonal balance and later impact fetal development
- **Genetic Factors:** Identifying variations that may affect hormone metabolism or reproductive function
- **Immune System Regulation:** Examining factors that could affect implantation and pregnancy maintenance

2. PERSONAL HISTORY ANALYSIS

Your health history contains vital clues about your fertility challenges:
- When did your reproductive symptoms begin?
- What other health challenges have you experienced?
- How have previous treatments affected your symptoms?
- What patterns have you noticed in your cycle, energy, digestion, or other functions?
- What environmental or emotional factors coincided with changes in your health?

3. LIFESTYLE EVALUATION

Daily habits and environmental factors significantly impact fertility:
- Nutrition patterns and food sensitivities
- Sleep quality and rhythm
- Stress levels and coping mechanisms
- Exercise type, intensity, and frequency
- Environmental exposures at home and work
- Personal care and household products
- Electronic device usage and EMF exposure

4. MEDICAL INTEGRATION

For optimal results, your fertility blueprint should integrate with appropriate medical care:
- Coordination with your reproductive endocrinologist if you're pursuing assisted reproduction
- Consideration of structural issues that may require surgical intervention
- Integration of therapeutic approaches for maximum effectiveness

- Clear communication between all healthcare providers involved in your care

Using all this information, we develop a customized fertility blueprint—a comprehensive plan addressing all factors affecting your reproductive health, from fundamental nutrition to specific supplement protocols, from stress management to medical treatments when needed.

This isn't a rigid blueprint but rather an adaptive design that evolves as your body responds to treatment. Like any good renovation project, we assess progress regularly, make necessary adjustments, and continue refining the approach until we achieve the desired outcome—a healthy pregnancy and baby.

THE RENOVATION TIMELINE: SETTING REALISTIC EXPECTATIONS

Before embarking on any home renovation, it's essential to understand the timeline. The same applies to your fertility renovation. While everyone's journey is unique, there are some general principles to keep in mind:

THE CELLULAR RENEWAL CYCLE

One of the most important concepts in fertility optimization is the time required for cellular renewal:

- **Egg Development:** The final maturation of an egg takes approximately 100 days (about 3 months)
- **Sperm Development:** Sperm develop over about 74 days (around 2.5 months)
- **Endometrial Lining:** Regenerates monthly with your cycle
- **Gut Lining:** Renews every 2–3 weeks

- **Liver Detoxification Capacity:** Can show improvements within weeks, but optimal function may take months to restore

This means that the dietary changes, supplements, and lifestyle modifications you implement today won't fully affect the eggs or sperm being released for at least 2-3 months. This is why patience and consistency are essential parts of the fertility renovation process. This is also why you should start this process as early as possible. However, I had my first child at 35 and my second at 40, demonstrating it is possible to start a family later in life. My journey was difficult, but I am so thankful to be where I am, and I promised myself and God that I would write this book when my family was complete. So here we are!

THE FUNCTIONAL MEDICINE TIMELINE

Based on my clinical experience and the research in functional medicine, here's a general timeline for fertility optimization:
- **1–2 months:** Initial detoxification, gut healing, and inflammation reduction
- **3–4 months:** Hormonal balance begins to improve, egg and sperm quality enhancement
- **4–6 months:** Optimal window for natural conception attempts or assisted reproductive technology
- **6+ months:** Continued optimization and adaptation based on response

For some people with mild imbalances, significant improvements may occur quickly. For others with more complex issues that may take time to discover and improve, the timeline may extend longer. Age is also a factor—older individuals may need more intensive intervention and support.

While this timeline may seem long if you're eager to conceive, remember that rushing the process rarely leads to optimal outcomes. Just as cutting corners in a home renovation often results in problems down the road, *skipping steps in your fertility optimization can lead to continued challenges or early pregnancy loss.*

BREAKING GROUND: WHERE TO BEGIN

Now that we understand the philosophy, the expanded heating/cooling metaphor, and the general approach to building your fertility blueprint, you might be wondering where to start. While your personal journey will be customized based on your specific needs, there are some fundamental steps almost everyone should take:

1. EXAMINE YOUR FOUNDATION

Just as we discussed in *Your Longevity Blueprint*, gut health forms the foundation of overall wellness, including reproductive health. Without a solid foundation, even the best climate control system won't function properly. Everything I shared in Chapter 1 of *Your Longevity Blueprint* regarding gut health applies here. In Chapter 18 of this book, we'll explore specific gut-fertility connections and protocols for optimization.

2. CHECK YOUR WIRING

Your neuroendocrine system—the communication network between your brain and hormonal glands—must function properly for reproductive hormones to stay balanced. Stress management, sleep optimization, and nervous system support form essential components of fertility renovation. We'll cover these in detail in later chapters.

3. ASSESS YOUR ENVIRONMENTAL INFLUENCES

External factors significantly impact your internal environment. Reducing exposure to endocrine-disrupting chemicals, electromagnetic fields, and other fertility-disrupting elements helps create a cleaner internal environment where conception can occur. Chapter 18 provides a comprehensive environmental optimization plan.

4. FOCUS ON YOUR CLIMATE CONTROL

With the fundamentals in place, we can fine-tune your hormonal system—addressing specific imbalances, optimizing feedback loops, and creating the perfect internal climate for conception. We will guide you through hormone-specific protocols.

5. CONSIDER STRUCTURAL REPAIRS

In some cases, physical issues may need correction—removing fibroids, addressing endometriosis, or repairing varicoceles, for example. We'll discuss when and how to incorporate these interventions into your overall fertility blueprint.

6. INTEGRATE CONVENTIONAL AND FUNCTIONAL APPROACHES

For many people, combining functional medicine optimization with conventional fertility treatments offers the best chance of success. We'll explore how to time these approaches for maximum effectiveness.

THE PROMISE OF THIS BLUEPRINT

As we conclude this introduction and prepare to dive into the specific systems affecting your fertility, I want to offer both hope and realism.

The functional medicine approach to fertility has helped thousands of people conceive healthy babies, even after years of failure with conventional treatments alone. By addressing the root causes of infertility rather than just managing the symptoms, we often see remarkable results.

Sarah, whose story I shared at the beginning, discovered that undiagnosed celiac disease was causing inflammatory immune reactions that led to her recurrent miscarriages. By removing gluten completely and healing her gut, she was able to conceive and carry a healthy pregnancy to term within six months.

Emma's testing revealed elevated natural killer cell activity and clotting factors that were affecting implantation. A protocol of immunomodulatory supplements, specialized nutrition, and low-dose blood thinners resulted in a successful pregnancy on her next attempt.

And Jennifer, who at 42 had been told donor eggs were her only option, embarked on a comprehensive four-month preparation protocol focusing on egg quality enhancement, inflammation reduction, and hormonal balance. She conceived naturally in her fifth cycle and delivered a healthy baby girl just before her 43rd birthday.

However, I must also acknowledge that not every fertility journey ends with a biological child. The functional medicine approach significantly improves your chances, but it cannot guarantee results, particularly in cases of advanced age or severe structural issues.

What I can promise is that following this blueprint will optimize your overall health, balance your hormones, and create the most fertile internal environment possible. These improvements benefit not just your reproductive health but your entire well-being—creating a solid foundation for whatever path your family-building journey ultimately takes.

This integrative approach ensures we're utilizing every evidence-based tool available to optimize your fertility. As we break ground on your fertility renovation, I invite you to approach the process with both determination and flexibility, trusting that each step brings you closer to hormonal balance and optimal health—*the best possible foundation for creating new life.*

My husband, Eric, will testify that I was one determined individual. He is forever thanking me for my relentless research, curiosity, and continued attempts down different paths to achieve our pregnancies. I do not take it for granted that God provided me the knowledge I needed in His timing, and I have deep conviction to share my journey with you to provide you hope that there are likely things your conventional provider hasn't even remotely considered that could be impairing your fertility.

In the next section, we'll explore the holistic impact of hormone balance on fertility, understanding how hormones affect and are affected by every dimension of your life—biological, psychological, social, cultural, spiritual. This integrative understanding forms the architectural framework upon which your entire fertility blueprint is built. Then we'll dive into a deeper understanding of our reproductive hormones.

SECTION II

STRUCTURAL INTEGRITY— THE HOLISTIC IMPACT OF HORMONE BALANCE ON FERTILITY

CHAPTER 4

THE FOUNDATION SYSTEMS—BIOLOGICAL AND PSYCHOLOGICAL ASPECTS OF FERTILITY

When we consider fertility challenges, it's easy to focus solely on the physical systems involved—examining hormone levels, evaluating reproductive organs, and targeting specific biological processes. However, just as a home is more than its foundation, plumbing, and electrical systems, human fertility encompasses dimensions far beyond biology alone.

In our home renovation metaphor, true structural integrity requires addressing every aspect of the building—from the foundation that supports it to the interior design that makes it livable, the family spaces that facilitate connection, the community context in which it exists, and even the sanctuary-like qualities that make it a true haven. Similarly, fertility health must be approached holistically, recognizing how hormonal balance affects and is affected by psychological, social, cultural, and spiritual dimensions.

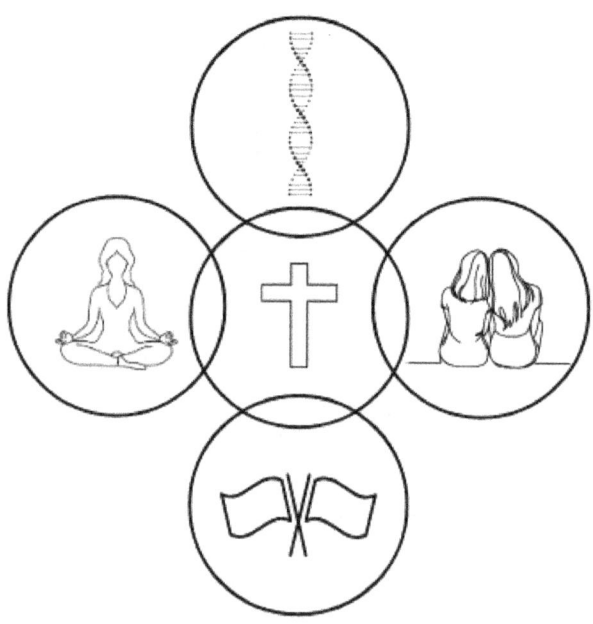

This section explores how hormone imbalances impact every aspect of life—and conversely, how these various dimensions of life influence our hormonal health. This holistic understanding is crucial for anyone seeking to optimize fertility, as it reveals both the far-reaching consequences of hormonal dysfunction and the multiple pathways through which healing can occur.

FOUNDATION STRENGTH: BIOLOGICAL FOUNDATIONS OF FERTILITY

Just as a home requires a solid foundation to withstand environmental stresses and support its structure, fertility depends on fundamental biological systems functioning in harmony. Hormone imbalances can compromise this foundation in profound and sometimes surprising ways.

THE INTERCONNECTED BIOLOGICAL SYSTEMS
THE REPRODUCTIVE-DIGESTIVE CONNECTION:

The digestive system plays a crucial role in hormonal health through several mechanisms:

- **Nutrient Absorption:** The gut must efficiently extract the building blocks needed for hormone production—proteins, healthy fats, vitamins, and minerals.
- **Estrogen Recycling:** The gut microbiome regulates estrogen levels through the "estrobolome"—bacterial genes that metabolize estrogens. Dysbiosis can lead to either estrogen deficiency or excess.
- **Inflammation Pathway:** Gut inflammation triggers systemic inflammation, which disrupts hormone signaling and egg/sperm quality.
- **Detoxification Support:** The intestinal lining helps eliminate hormone-disrupting chemicals and excess hormones.

When hormone imbalances exist, they often manifest in digestive symptoms:

- PMS-related bloating and constipation
- Estrogen-dominant diarrhea
- Thyroid-related digestive slowing
- Cortisol-triggered irritable bowel symptoms

THE REPRODUCTIVE-IMMUNE INTERFACE:

The immune system and reproductive system share a complex relationship:

- **Immune Tolerance:** Successful pregnancy requires the immune system to tolerate the "foreign" genetic material of

the embryo—a process regulated by hormones, particularly progesterone.
- **Autoimmunity Connection:** Hormonal fluctuations can trigger or suppress autoimmune conditions. Conversely, autoimmune conditions (like celiac or antiphospholipid syndrome) often correlate with infertility and pregnancy complications.
- **Inflammation Impact:** Chronic inflammation can damage egg and sperm quality while also disrupting hormone receptors and signaling.
- **Infection Response:** The reproductive tract's immune defense against infections is influenced by hormone levels, with estrogen generally enhancing immunity and progesterone modulating it.

Hormonal imbalances frequently manifest in immune dysfunction:
- Increased susceptibility to vaginal and urinary infections
- Heightened inflammatory responses
- Autoimmune flares with cycle changes
- Recurrent pregnancy loss due to immune dysregulation

THE REPRODUCTIVE-NEUROLOGICAL AXIS:

The brain and reproductive system maintain constant communication:
- **Hypothalamic Control:** The hypothalamus serves as the master controller of reproduction, sensing environmental conditions and initiating hormonal cascades.
- **Feedback Loops:** Neurological circuits monitor hormone levels and adjust signaling accordingly.

- **Neurotransmitter Overlap:** Many neurological messengers such as serotonin, dopamine, and gamma-aminobutyric acid (GABA) also influence reproductive function.
- **Pain Processing:** Hormone fluctuations affect pain perception, particularly in reproductive organs.

Hormone imbalances often create neurological symptoms:
- Cycle-related migraines
- Premenstrual mood changes
- Menopause-related cognitive changes
- PCOS-associated anxiety

THE REPRODUCTIVE-METABOLIC CONNECTION:

Energy metabolism and reproduction are fundamentally linked:
- **Insulin Signaling:** Insulin resistance directly affects ovarian function and is central to PCOS pathology.
- **Fat Cell Activity:** Adipose tissue produces estrogen and inflammatory compounds that influence fertility.
- **Metabolic Rate:** Thyroid function affects both metabolism and reproductive hormone balance.
- **Energy Allocation:** The body prioritizes survival over reproduction when energy is scarce.

Hormone imbalances frequently disrupt metabolism:
- PCOS-related weight challenges
- Estrogen-dominant fat distribution changes
- Hypothyroid-related metabolic slowing
- Cortisol-driven abdominal weight gain

THE FOUNDATION'S HIDDEN CRACKS: SUBCLINICAL DEFICIENCIES

Just as a home's foundation may contain invisible cracks that only reveal themselves during stress, many hormonal imbalances remain subclinical—not severe enough to trigger a medical diagnosis but sufficient to compromise fertility and well-being.

COMMON SUBCLINICAL DEFICIENCIES:

- **Thyroid Function:** Even "normal range" thyroid values can be suboptimal for fertility, with TSH above 2.5 mIU/L associated with reduced conception rates and increased miscarriage. I can't tell you how many patients I treated and ALL I did was optimize their thyroid and they conceived—and when I say optimize, I mean improved their T3 (more on that later).

- **Vitamin D Status:** Levels below 40 ng/mL may impact fertility, though they're not flagged as deficient in standard testing.

- **Luteal Phase Deficiency:** Subtle progesterone insufficiency may not prevent ovulation but can compromise implantation and early pregnancy maintenance. Progesterone is something I have taken for years, and even required it through my pregnancies. Beyond optimizing T3, optimizing progesterone has also helped countless women in my practice achieve and maintain pregnancies. Simply monitoring progesterone through pregnancy is extremely valuable and something that, even if monitored in conventional medicine during the first trimester, rarely continues after. When I hear stories of second-trimester losses, my heart sinks, and I always wonder if progesterone could have helped.

- **Functional Hypercortisolism:** Stress-induced cortisol patterns can disrupt other hormones without meeting criteria for Cushing's syndrome.

- **Borderline Testosterone Levels:** Levels may not qualify as a clinical deficiency but are insufficient to support optimal libido, energy, and egg/sperm quality.

The functional medicine approach emphasizes identifying and addressing these foundation cracks before they compromise the entire structure—restoring optimal hormone function rather than merely treating disease states.

THE BIOLOGICAL REPAIR PROCESS

Restoring biological foundation strength involves a systematic approach:

1. **Assessment:** Comprehensive testing to identify both obvious and subtle imbalances
2. **Nutritional Reinforcement:** Providing the raw materials needed for hormone production and metabolism, as well as egg and sperm quality
3. **Detoxification Support:** Removing hormone-disrupting chemicals and supporting healthy hormone clearance
4. **Inflammation Reduction:** Addressing sources of chronic inflammation that disrupt hormone signaling
5. **Gut Repair:** Restoring microbiome diversity and intestinal integrity

6. **Hormonal Support:** Strategic use of bioidentical hormones or herbal adaptogens when indicated
7. **Metabolic Optimization:** Improving insulin sensitivity and energy regulation

By strengthening these biological foundations, we create the physical capacity for fertility while simultaneously enhancing overall health—similar to how reinforcing a home's foundation improves not just structural integrity but also the function and longevity of all other components.

INTERIOR DESIGN: PSYCHOLOGICAL ASPECTS OF THE FERTILITY JOURNEY

Just as a home's interior design affects how we experience and function within the space, our psychological state profoundly influences—and is influenced by—our hormonal health and fertility. The mind-body connection represents one of the most powerful yet often overlooked aspects of reproductive wellness.

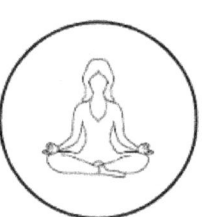

THE HORMONE-EMOTION CYCLE
Hormones and emotions exist in a continuous feedback loop:

HOW HORMONES SHAPE EMOTIONS:
- **Estrogen:** Enhances serotonin and dopamine activity, generally improving mood, motivation, and verbal memory when balanced

- **Progesterone:** Exerts calming effects through GABA modulation, reducing anxiety when optimal but potentially causing mood changes when fluctuating
- **Testosterone:** Influences confidence, assertiveness, and libido in both men and women
- **Cortisol:** Acute elevation increases alertness and focus, while chronic elevation triggers anxiety and depression
- **Thyroid Hormones:** Regulate energy, motivation, and cognitive processing speed
- **Oxytocin:** Promotes bonding, trust, and stress reduction

HOW EMOTIONS SHAPE HORMONES:

- **Chronic Stress:** Elevates cortisol, which can suppress reproductive hormone production
- **Depression:** Often correlates with lower dopamine and serotonin, which affects hypothalamic-pituitary signaling
- **Anxiety:** Activates sympathetic nervous system, diverting resources away from reproductive function
- **Grief:** Can trigger inflammatory responses that disrupt hormone balance
- **Joy and Connection:** Promote parasympathetic "rest and digest" state conducive to reproductive function
- **Security and Safety:** Support optimal hypothalamic function and hormone pulsatility

This bidirectional relationship explains why fertility challenges often involve both psychological and hormonal components that must be addressed simultaneously—like renovating a home's layout while also addressing the emotional associations with each space.

THE PSYCHOLOGICAL IMPACT OF FERTILITY CHALLENGES

Hormone imbalances and fertility difficulties create significant psychological burdens:

- **Identity Disruption:** Infertility can challenge core aspects of self-concept and life expectations
- **Relationship Strain:** Sexual timing, treatment decisions, and grief can stress partnerships
- **Anxiety and Control:** The uncertainty of fertility outcomes can trigger profound anxiety
- **Grief Cycles:** Each unsuccessful attempt or loss initiates a grief process
- **Social Isolation:** Feeling disconnected from peers who conceive easily
- **Treatment Trauma:** Medical interventions can be physically and emotionally traumatic
- **Financial Stress:** The cost of treatments adds significant pressure

The conventional medical approach often focuses solely on biological interventions while overlooking these psychological dimensions—similar to renovating a home's systems without considering how the residents will live within the space.

PSYCHOLOGICAL RENOVATION STRATEGIES

The functional medicine approach integrates psychological healing into fertility treatment:

1. **Stress Physiology Management:**
    - Mind-body practices (meditation, yoga, breathwork)
    - Heart rate variability training
    - Sleep optimization protocols

- Nature exposure and grounding practices
- Strategic exercise appropriate to hormonal state

2. **Emotional Processing Support:**
   - Trauma-informed therapy modalities
   - Grief work for pregnancy loss or fertility disappointments
   - Cognitive approaches for anxiety and rumination
   - Somatic practices for embodied stress release
   - Creative expression of fertility emotions

3. **Relationship Strengthening:**
   - Communication tools for fertility discussions
   - Preserving intimacy beyond conception timing
   - Shared decision-making frameworks
   - Partner inclusion in the fertility process
   - Maintaining connection through treatment challenges

4. **Identity and Purpose Work:**
   - Exploring self-concept beyond reproduction
   - Finding meaning in the fertility journey itself
   - Developing flexible visions of family creation
   - Community contribution and legacy building
   - Integrating fertility challenges into life narrative

5. **Neurotransmitter Support:**
   - Nutritional precursors for mood-regulating neurotransmitters
   - Targeted amino acid therapy
   - Herbal adaptogens for stress resilience
   - Anti-inflammatory approaches for brain health
   - Gut-brain axis optimization

By addressing these psychological aspects of fertility, we not only improve quality of life during the fertility journey but also optimize the hormonal environment for conception—creating an interior design that supports both well-being and functionality.

CHAPTER 5

THE SOCIAL ARCHITECTURE—FAMILY DYNAMICS AND CULTURAL CONTEXT IN FERTILITY

FAMILY SPACES: SOCIAL DIMENSIONS OF REPRODUCTIVE HEALTH

Just as a home includes spaces specifically designed for family gathering and connection, fertility exists within a social context that significantly influences reproductive outcomes. Hormone balance affects, and is affected by, our relationships, support systems, and social functioning.

THE SOCIAL-HORMONAL CONNECTION

Social interactions trigger powerful hormonal responses:
- **Oxytocin Release:** Physical touch, emotional intimacy, and social bonding trigger oxytocin, which modulates stress response and supports reproductive function

- **Stress Buffer Effect:** Strong social support reduces cortisol reactivity to stressors
- **Cycle Synchronization:** Women living together often experience menstrual synchrony through pheromonal communication
- **Social Rank Influences:** Perceived social status affects testosterone and cortisol patterns
- **Belonging Impact:** Social connection promotes parasympathetic nervous system activation conducive to fertility

Conversely, hormone imbalances can profoundly affect social functioning:

- **Estrogen Fluctuations:** Affect verbal fluency, empathy, and social sensitivity
- **Testosterone Variations:** Influence assertiveness, competition, and social confidence
- **Progesterone Shifts:** Alter desire for social contact and emotional responses to others
- **Cortisol Dysregulation:** Can trigger social withdrawal or conflict sensitivity
- **Thyroid Imbalances:** May cause social fatigue or anxiety in group settings

This reciprocal relationship means that fertility support must consider the social environment—just as home design must account for how family members interact within shared spaces.

SOCIAL CHALLENGES OF THE FERTILITY JOURNEY

The fertility path often creates unique social difficulties:

- **Celebration Avoidance:** Difficulty attending baby showers, birthdays, or family gatherings
- **Advice Overload:** Managing unsolicited suggestions from well-meaning friends and family
- **Comparison Triggers:** Social media and peer milestones intensifying feelings of inadequacy
- **Disclosure Decisions:** Navigating privacy versus support needs
- **Support Disparities:** Friends and family who don't understand fertility challenges
- **Work-Treatment Conflicts:** Balancing career demands with appointment schedules
- **Financial-Social Tradeoffs:** Treatment costs limiting social participation

These challenges can trigger stress responses that further compromise hormone balance—creating a negative cycle that affects fertility outcomes.

SOCIAL SPACE RENOVATION

Optimizing the social dimension of fertility involves intentional strategies:

1. **Curating Supportive Environments:**
    - Setting boundaries with triggering situations or relationships
    - Cultivating relationships with those who understand fertility challenges

- Joining fertility support communities (in-person or online)
- Creating rituals for processing difficult social events
- Developing scripts for handling intrusive questions

2. **Partner Relationship Enhancement:**
   - Scheduled connection time unrelated to fertility
   - Shared self-care practices
   - Division of emotional labor in the fertility process
   - Honoring different coping styles and grief expressions
   - Maintaining physical intimacy beyond conception attempts

3. **Communication Blueprints:**
   - Clear boundaries with family about fertility discussions
   - Educated responses to misinformation or simplistic advice
   - Vulnerability with selected support people
   - Explicit requests for specific types of support
   - Fertility-friendly language and metaphors

4. **Social Hormone Optimization:**
   - Regular meaningful connection to boost oxytocin
   - Laughter and play to reduce stress hormones
   - Physical touch (partner, pets, massage) for hormonal regulation
   - Group activities that promote belonging and purpose
   - Balancing solitude and social time based on hormonal fluctuations

By thoughtfully designing the social environment, individuals and couples can create spaces that support rather than hinder hormonal balance—much like thoughtfully designed family spaces in a home that facilitate connection while respecting individual needs.

COMMUNITY PLANNING: CULTURAL INFLUENCES ON FERTILITY DECISIONS

Just as a home exists within a neighborhood and community that shapes its accessibility, value, and function, fertility decisions take place within cultural contexts that profoundly influence reproductive choices, timing, and approaches to challenges. These cultural factors interact with biological systems, sometimes supporting and sometimes hindering hormonal health.

THE CULTURAL-HORMONAL INTERFACE

Cultural norms and expectations create physiological responses:

- **Fertility Timelines:** Cultural expectations about appropriate ages for childbearing create psychological pressure that can affect hormone regulation
- **Success Definitions:** Cultural messages about career achievement versus family formation influence life planning and stress physiology
- **Body Ideals:** Cultural standards of attractiveness affect body image, eating patterns, and resulting hormonal function
- **Gender Expectations:** Cultural gender roles shape stress responses, relationship dynamics, and approaches to fertility challenges

- **Medical Trust:** Cultural attitudes toward conventional versus traditional medicine influence treatment choices and nocebo/placebo responses
- **Family Size Norms:** Cultural expectations about family size create pressure that affects fertility decisions and treatments

These cultural factors don't just influence decisions—they create physiological responses that directly impact hormone function and fertility outcomes.

THE WEIGHT OF CULTURAL EXPECTATIONS: A PERSONAL MOMENT

I remember sitting in church a few years ago, right after an early loss following IVF…on Mother's Day, of all days. The family in front of me took up an entire row with their children—I counted literally nine kids ranging from toddlers to teenagers. While I wanted to feel joy for their obvious blessings, all I could feel was the weight of my own empty arms and the cultural message that seemed to scream around me: that having one child somehow wasn't enough, that I wasn't complete as a woman or fulfilling my purpose as a wife.

It felt like everyone around me kept effortlessly expanding their families while I fought tooth and nail for each pregnancy attempt. The cultural pressure was suffocating—the subtle comments about giving William a sibling, the assumptions that we'd naturally have more children, the way conversations seemed to revolve around family size as a measure of success or blessing. In that church seat, feeling physically and emotionally depleted from our recent loss, I felt like I was failing at the most fundamental expectation placed on women.

Man, was I trying though. But it didn't seem fair that she kept getting pregnant and I didn't. The comparison game became toxic, and

I found myself avoiding social gatherings where I knew there would be pregnancy announcements or discussions about growing families.

Here's what I want you to know if you're in a similar place: it's okay to struggle with others' good news when you're in the thick of your own battle. That doesn't make you a bad person—it makes you human. But your story isn't over. Your journey matters. And sometimes, the path to parenthood looks different from what we expected—but that doesn't mean it's not meant for you.

CONTEMPORARY CULTURAL CHALLENGES TO FERTILITY

Several aspects of modern culture particularly impact reproductive health:

- **Delayed Childbearing:** Career development often pushes reproduction to advanced maternal age, when hormone production naturally declines
- **Environmental Exposures:** Industrialized living introduces numerous hormone-disrupting chemicals
- **Digital Disruption:** Screen time and artificial light alter melatonin production, which coordinates reproductive hormones
- **Disconnect from Nature:** Separation from natural environments and cycles disrupts hormonal entrainment
- **Productivity Pressure:** Cultural emphasis on constant productivity creates chronic stress patterns
- **Medicalization of Reproduction:** Technological approaches sometimes bypass rather than address underlying hormonal imbalances
- **Nutrition Transitions:** Modern food systems provide caloric abundance but micronutrient scarcity

The conventional approach often fails to acknowledge these cultural influences, treating fertility as purely biological—similar to designing a home without considering the neighborhood context, available resources, or community needs.

CULTURAL RENOVATION APPROACHES

A functional medicine perspective recognizes and addresses these cultural dimensions:

1. **Conscious Cultural Navigation:**
    - Identifying internalized beliefs about fertility and family
    - Distinguishing personal values from cultural pressures
    - Creating intentional timelines based on biological realities
    - Developing language for discussing fertility choices with family and community
    - Finding cultural subgroups that support your reproductive values

2. **Environmental Hormone Protection:**
    - Creating clean living spaces with minimal endocrine disruptors
    - Choosing low-toxic personal care and cleaning products
    - Filtering water and air to reduce chemical exposures
    - Selecting hormone-supportive food sources
    - Advocating for community-level environmental protections

3. **Circadian Rhythm Restoration:**
   - Morning sunlight exposure to regulate hormone pulsatility
   - Evening blue light reduction to support melatonin production
   - Technology boundaries that respect biological rhythms
   - Seasonal awareness and adjustment of activities
   - Meal timing aligned with metabolic and hormonal patterns

4. **Nature Connection Practices:**
   - Regular immersion in natural environments
   - Observation of natural fertility cycles in ecosystems
   - Barefoot contact with earth (grounding)
   - Alignment with lunar cycles (which often correlate with menstrual patterns)
   - Incorporation of natural elements into home environment

5. **Cultural Resource Integration:**
   - Identifying supportive aspects of personal cultural heritage
   - Incorporating traditional wisdom about fertility when evidence-supported
   - Creating community rituals for fertility journey milestones
   - Exploring culturally resonant mind-body practices
   - Finding meaning frameworks within cultural or spiritual traditions

By consciously engaging with cultural influences rather than simply being shaped by them, individuals can create environments more conducive to hormonal health—similar to how thoughtful community planning creates neighborhoods that support rather than undermine the function and value of individual homes.

CHAPTER 6

CREATING SACRED SPACE—SPIRITUAL DIMENSIONS OF THE FERTILITY JOURNEY

SANCTUARY DESIGN: SPIRITUAL ASPECTS OF CREATING LIFE

Just as the most beloved homes contain elements that transcend mere functionality to create a sense of sanctuary and meaning, the fertility journey has profound spiritual dimensions that affect and are affected by hormonal health. Creating life—or facing challenges in doing so—inevitably raises questions about purpose, meaning, and connection to something larger than ourselves.

THE SPIRITUAL-HORMONAL CONNECTION

Spiritual states create physiological responses that influence hormone balance:

- **Awe and Wonder:** Experiences of awe reduce inflammatory markers and regulate stress hormones

- **Purpose and Meaning:** A sense of purpose improves hypothalamic-pituitary-adrenal axis regulation
- **Surrender and Acceptance:** Releasing control reduces chronic cortisol elevation
- **Gratitude Practice:** Appreciation activities improve parasympathetic nervous system function
- **Connection to Larger Reality:** Transcendent experiences promote integrated nervous system regulation
- **Compassion Cultivation:** Self-compassion improves oxytocin release and stress recovery

Conversely, spiritual struggles can compromise hormone balance:
- **Existential Questioning:** Uncertainty about meaning can increase anxiety physiology
- **Reproductive Grief:** Loss and disappointment can trigger inflammatory responses
- **Faith Community Challenges:** Religious communities can be either supportive or triggering
- **Purpose Disruption:** Fertility challenges may undermine sense of life purpose
- **Body-Spirit Disconnect:** Feeling betrayed by one's body can create stress responses
- **Worthiness Wounds:** Questioning one's deservingness can affect hormone regulation

These connections highlight why addressing spiritual dimensions is not supplemental but essential to hormonal health—just as creating sanctuary aspects in a home is not merely decorative but fundamental to its function as a nurturing space.

SPIRITUAL CHALLENGES OF FERTILITY

The fertility journey often triggers profound spiritual questions:
- **Why Me?:** Questioning why fertility challenges are happening
- **Deservingness:** Wrestling with feelings of undeservingness or punishment
- **Body Trust:** Struggling to trust a body that isn't functioning as expected
- **Control Illusion:** Confronting the limits of control over life creation
- **Meaning Making:** Finding purpose in the suffering of fertility struggles
- **Legacy Concerns:** Questioning how to create meaning and legacy
- **Divine Relationship:** Navigating feelings toward God or higher power
- **Life Transition:** Moving between identity stages without clear rituals

Conventional approaches rarely address these spiritual dimensions, focusing instead on technological solutions—similar to renovating a home's systems without attending to the elements that create a sense of sanctuary and belonging.

SANCTUARY CREATION STRATEGIES

A holistic approach integrates spiritual support into fertility care:
1. **Meaning-Making Practices:**
    - Journaling about the personal meaning of the fertility journey

- Creating rituals to honor losses and transitions
- Identifying growth and wisdom emerging from challenges
- Connecting personal story to archetypal or traditional narratives
- Finding purpose beyond biological reproduction

2. **Body-Spirit Reconnection:**
   - Somatic practices that foster embodied presence
   - Blessing or gratitude rituals for the body regardless of function
   - Movement practices that celebrate the body's capabilities
   - Visualization of harmony between physical and spiritual aspects

3. **Transcendent Connection:**
   - Time in natural settings that evoke awe
   - Meditation practices that expand self-concept beyond physical body
   - Prayer or intention-setting aligned with personal beliefs
   - Community experiences that create belonging to something larger
   - Creative expression that channels fertility emotions into meaningful form

4. **Wisdom Tradition Resources:**
   - Exploring fertility-related teachings from personal spiritual background

- Studying cross-cultural approaches to reproduction and meaning
- Connecting with spiritual leaders who understand fertility challenges
- Adapting traditional rituals for contemporary fertility journeys
- Finding fertility-supportive communities within wisdom traditions

5. **Legacy Beyond Biology:**
   - Mentoring or teaching relationships that create non-biological legacy
   - Creative works that express unique gifts and perspective
   - Community contribution that makes meaningful impact
   - Environmental stewardship as care for future generations
   - Family connection that transcends genetic relationships

By nurturing these spiritual dimensions, individuals create internal sanctuary spaces that support hormonal balance through difficult fertility terrain—much like how thoughtfully designed sanctuary elements in a home provide resilience through life's challenges.

BIBLICAL WISDOM: ANCIENT FERTILITY JOURNEYS

The struggle with fertility is as old as humanity itself, and the Bible contains several profound stories of women whose fertility journeys offer timeless wisdom and comfort. Sarah, Abraham's

wife, laughed in disbelief when told she would bear a child in her nineties—yet her story became one of miraculous fulfillment despite advanced age. Rachel cried out, "Give me children, or I shall die!" expressing the raw anguish that many women still feel today, before eventually conceiving Joseph. Hannah prayed so fervently for a child that she was mistaken for being drunk, her lips moving silently in desperate prayer—a prayer that was ultimately answered with the birth of Samuel, whom she dedicated to God in gratitude.

Elizabeth, the mother of John the Baptist, endured years of what the Bible calls "barrenness" and the accompanying social shame, only to conceive in her older years. And Ruth's story reminds us of the importance of community and family support during reproductive challenges. These women's journeys reveal several spiritual principles relevant to fertility today: the importance of persistent **hope** even when circumstances seem impossible; the power of honest emotional expression; the value of prayer and faith during waiting periods; and the understanding that fertility journeys often have timing beyond our control.

What's particularly striking about these biblical accounts is that they don't gloss over the emotional and spiritual struggles these women faced. They acknowledged anger, jealousy, grief, and questioning. They sometimes took matters into their own hands before surrendering to a higher plan. And importantly, their worth and purpose were ultimately affirmed regardless of their reproductive status—a powerful reminder for those on similar journeys today.

These ancient stories remind us that while our scientific understanding of fertility has advanced tremendously, the emotional and spiritual dimensions of creating life remain remarkably consistent across millennia. They offer a sacred connection to countless generations of women who have walked similar paths before us, creating a sense of timeless community around an experience that can often feel isolating in our modern world.

THE HOLISTIC BLUEPRINT: INTEGRATING ALL DIMENSIONS

True structural integrity in both homes and hormonal health requires integration of all dimensions. Just as a well-designed home considers foundation, interior design, family spaces, community context, and sanctuary elements as an integrated whole, optimal fertility support addresses **biological, psychological, social, cultural, and spiritual** aspects as interconnected facets of health.

The functional medicine approach recognizes this integration through several key principles:

1. **Multidirectional Influence:** Each dimension affects all others, creating both challenges and multiple entry points for healing.
2. **Individualized Design:** Just as each home renovation must respect the unique structure and needs of the building, fertility support must be tailored to individual values, circumstances, and biology.
3. **Systems Thinking:** Both homes and bodies function as integrated systems where changing one element affects all others.
4. **Both/And Approach:** Technological interventions AND lifestyle modifications, physical healing AND emotional processing, individual optimization AND relationship nurturing are all essential.
5. **Process Orientation:** Both home renovation and fertility health involve ongoing adaptation rather than one-time fixes.

In the chapters that follow, we'll explore specific structural challenges that affect fertility—from endometriosis to PCOS, from male factor issues to unexplained infertility—always remembering that these conditions affect and are affected by all dimensions of human experience. By maintaining this holistic perspective, we create the opportunity for deeper healing that extends far beyond reproductive function alone—much like how a thoughtful home renovation improves not just the building's integrity but the entire lived experience of its inhabitants.

Just as the most successful home renovations honor both the physical structure and the human needs it serves, the most effective fertility support honors both the biological processes of reproduction and the whole-person experience of creating life.

As my Christian faith is a huge part of my life and thus my fertility journey, as I conclude this section, I'd like to share a prayer with you to use and to read over yourself daily as you continue this book and his journey.

A PRAYER FOR YOUR FERTILITY JOURNEY

This prayer can be used during moments of reflection, struggle,
or hope throughout your fertility journey.

Dear Heavenly Father,

    Creator of all life, I come before You with both my hopes and my heartaches on this fertility journey. You formed each of us with intricate care, knitting us together in our mothers' wombs, and I trust that You see and know every cell of my body and every longing of my heart.

    Lord, I ask for Your healing touch on my body. Where there is imbalance, bring harmony. Where there is inflammation, bring peace. Where there is dysfunction, restore Your perfect design. Let every system work as You intended, from the deepest cellular processes to the complex dance of hormones that sustains life.

    Grant wisdom to my healthcare providers. Guide their minds to see beyond symptoms to root causes. Direct my path to the right treatments, interventions, and supportive care. When I face decisions, illuminate the way that leads to wholeness and life.

Father, strengthen me emotionally for this journey. On days when disappointment weighs heavy, be my comfort. When anxiety rises, be my peace. When waiting seems endless, be my patience. Help me remain present in each day rather than losing today's blessings to tomorrow's worries.

I pray for my relationship with my partner/spouse, that this journey would bring us closer rather than pulling us apart. Help us communicate with honesty and tenderness, supporting each other through every high and low.

Lord, I surrender my timeline to You, trusting that Your timing is perfect even when I don't understand. I release my grip on control, knowing that while I can take steps toward healing, ultimately new life comes from You alone.

If it is Your will, bless us with a child. Prepare our home, our hearts, and our bodies to nurture new life. And if our path to parenthood looks different from what we imagined, give us the courage and clarity to follow where You lead.

Thank You for walking alongside me through every test, treatment, hope, and heartbreak. Thank You for Your promise to work all things together for good for those who love You. I choose to trust You today with both my fertility and my future.

In Your holy name I pray,
Amen.

"For I know the plans I have for you," declares the LORD, "plans to prosper you and not to harm you, plans to give you hope and a future."
— Jeremiah 29:11

"Hope deferred makes the heart sick, but a longing fulfilled is a tree of life."
— Proverbs 13:12

"But they that wait upon the LORD shall renew their strength; they shall mount up with wings as eagles; they shall run, and not be weary; and they shall walk, and not faint."
— Isaiah 40:31

SECTION III

ENGINEERING THE SYSTEMS—UNDERSTANDING REPRODUCTIVE HORMONES

CHAPTER 7

SYSTEM ARCHITECTURE— ANATOMY AND CLIMATE CONTROL

UNDERSTANDING YOUR REPRODUCTIVE HOME: THE ESSENTIAL SYSTEMS (ANATOMY REVIEW)

Before we explore the complex hormonal engineering that controls fertility, it's important to understand the physical structures that make up your reproductive home. Just as you need to know the layout of a house before renovating it, understanding reproductive anatomy helps you appreciate how the functional medicine approaches in this book optimize each component of your fertility system.

Think of your reproductive anatomy as a specialized home designed for one ultimate purpose: creating and nurturing new life. Like any well-designed home, each room and system has a specific function, and all components must work together harmoniously for optimal performance.

THE FEMALE REPRODUCTIVE HOME
THE OVARIES: PRODUCTION FACILITIES

Your ovaries function as the primary production facilities of your reproductive home, manufacturing both eggs and the hormones that orchestrate your entire fertility cycle.

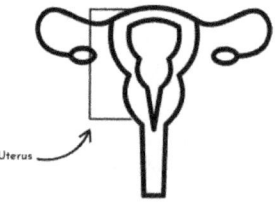

Structure and Location:
- Two almond-sized organs located on either side of the uterus
- Connected to the uterus by the fallopian tubes
- Contain all the eggs you'll ever have (present since before birth)

Key Functions:
- **Egg Storage and Maturation:** House approximately 1–2 million eggs at birth, decreasing to about 300,000–400,000 by puberty
- **Hormone Production:** Manufacture estrogen, progesterone, and small amounts of testosterone
- **Monthly Ovulation:** Release mature eggs for potential fertilization
- **Cycle Regulation:** Respond to brain signals (FSH and LH) to coordinate reproductive timing

THE FALLOPIAN TUBES: TRANSPORT CORRIDORS

The fallopian tubes serve as sophisticated transport corridors, designed to capture eggs and provide the optimal environment for fertilization.

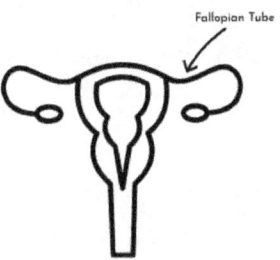

Structure and Function:
- Two narrow tubes (about four inches long) extending from each ovary to the uterus
- Lined with tiny hair-like projections (cilia) that create gentle currents
- Widened ends (fimbriae) that sweep over the ovaries to capture released eggs

Critical Roles:
- **Egg Capture:** Fimbriae collect the egg after ovulation
- **Fertilization Site:** Where sperm typically meets egg
- **Embryo Transport:** Cilia move the developing embryo toward the uterus
- **Nutrient Provision:** Provide nourishment for the early embryo during its 5–6 day journey

THE UTERUS: THE NURTURING CHAMBER

Your uterus is the ultimate nurturing chamber—a remarkable organ designed to house and support a growing baby for nine months.

Structure:
- **Fundus:** The upper portion where embryos typically implant
- **Body:** The main chamber that expands during pregnancy
- **Cervix:** The lower opening that connects to the vagina
- **Endometrium:** The inner lining that thickens and sheds with each cycle
- **Myometrium:** The muscular wall that contracts during menstruation and labor

Essential Functions:
- **Implantation Site:** Provides the location where embryos attach and begin developing
- **Nutrient Supply:** Rich blood supply nourishes the developing baby
- **Protection:** Muscular walls and amniotic fluid protect the growing fetus
- **Delivery Mechanism:** Powerful contractions help deliver the baby

THE CERVIX: THE GATEWAY GUARDIAN

The cervix functions as an intelligent gateway, regulating what enters and exits the uterus throughout your cycle.

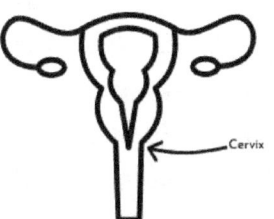

Remarkable Capabilities:
- **Mucus Production:** Creates different types of cervical mucus throughout the cycle
- **Sperm Filter:** Allows healthy sperm passage while blocking debris and bacteria
- **Pregnancy Protection:** Forms a mucus plug during pregnancy to protect the developing baby
- **Delivery Preparation:** Softens and dilates during labor to allow birth

Supporting Structures:
- **The Vagina:** The welcoming entrance to your reproductive home, designed to receive sperm and provide an exit pathway for menstrual flow and birth.
- **The Vulva:** The external structures that protect the internal reproductive organs, including the labia, clitoris, and vaginal opening.

THE MALE REPRODUCTIVE HOME
THE TESTES: MANUFACTURING CENTERS

The testes function as highly specialized manufacturing centers, producing both sperm and the hormones essential for male fertility.

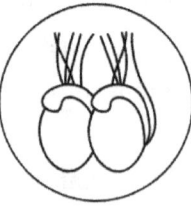

Structure and Location:
- Two oval-shaped organs housed in the scrotum
- Located outside the body to maintain optimal temperature for sperm production
- Connected to internal structures through the spermatic cord

Critical Functions:
- **Sperm Production:** Manufacture approximately 300 million sperm daily
- **Hormone Production:** Primary source of testosterone and other male hormones
- **Temperature Regulation:** Maintain the 2–4 degree temperature difference needed for healthy sperm development

THE EPIDIDYMIS: MATURATION AND STORAGE FACILITIES

- **Structure:** Coiled tubes attached to each testis
- **Function:** Sperm mature and gain motility during their 2–3 week journey through these tubes
- **Storage:** Mature sperm are stored here until ejaculation

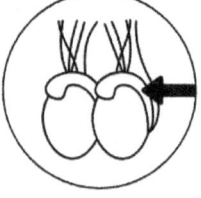

THE VAS DEFERENS: TRANSPORT HIGHWAYS
- **Structure:** Two long tubes that transport sperm from the epididymis to the urethra
- **Function:** Muscular contractions propel sperm during ejaculation
- **Strategic Importance:** Can be blocked by infection, injury, or surgical procedures

THE ACCESSORY GLANDS: SUPPORT SYSTEMS
SEMINAL VESICLES:
- Produce fructose-rich fluid that provides energy for sperm
- Contribute approximately 60% of seminal fluid volume

PROSTATE GLAND:
- Produces alkaline fluid that neutralizes vaginal acidity
- Contains enzymes that help sperm mobility
- Contributes about 30% of seminal fluid

BULBOURETHRAL GLANDS:
- Produce pre-ejaculatory fluid that neutralizes urethral acidity
- Clear the urethral pathway for sperm passage

HOW THE SYSTEMS WORK TOGETHER
THE MONTHLY COORDINATION (FEMALE)
Your reproductive anatomy operates on a precisely timed monthly schedule:

1. **Follicular Phase:** Ovaries prepare eggs while the uterus rebuilds its lining
2. **Ovulation:** Mature egg travels from ovary through fallopian tube
3. **Luteal Phase:** Uterus maintains its lining while waiting for potential pregnancy
4. **Menstruation:** If no pregnancy occurs, the uterine lining sheds and the cycle begins again

THE CONTINUOUS PRODUCTION (MALE)

Male reproductive anatomy works on a continuous production schedule:

1. **Sperm Creation:** Testes continuously produce new sperm (74-day cycle from start to maturity)
2. **Maturation Process:** Sperm gain motility and functionality in the epididymis
3. **Storage and Preparation:** Mature sperm await ejaculation while accessory glands prepare supportive fluids
4. **Delivery System:** During ejaculation, sperm mix with seminal fluid and travel through the reproductive tract

THE CONCEPTION PROCESS: WHEN SYSTEMS UNITE

Understanding how male and female reproductive anatomy work together during conception helps illustrate why optimal function of all systems is crucial:

1. **Sperm Delivery:** During intercourse, sperm are deposited in the vagina
2. **Cervical Navigation:** Healthy sperm swim through cervical mucus (quality depends on hormonal balance)

3. **Uterine Journey:** Sperm travel through the uterus toward the fallopian tubes
4. **Fertilization:** If an egg is present, fertilization typically occurs in the fallopian tube
5. **Embryo Development:** The fertilized egg begins dividing while traveling toward the uterus
6. **Implantation:** The embryo attaches to the prepared uterine lining
7. **Early Pregnancy:** Hormonal changes support the developing pregnancy

WHY ANATOMY MATTERS FOR FUNCTIONAL MEDICINE

Understanding reproductive anatomy is crucial for appreciating how functional medicine approaches enhance fertility:

Hormonal Integration: Every structure depends on proper hormonal signaling to function optimally. When we balance hormones through nutrition, supplements, and lifestyle changes, we're optimizing the function of these physical structures.

Blood Flow Requirements: All reproductive organs require excellent circulation to function properly. The detoxification, exercise, and stress-reduction strategies in this book enhance blood flow to these critical areas.

Inflammation Impact: Chronic inflammation can affect every aspect of reproductive anatomy, from egg quality in the ovaries to sperm production in the testes to implantation in the uterus.

Environmental Sensitivity: Reproductive organs are particularly sensitive to environmental toxins, making the environmental cleanup strategies in this book essential for optimal function.

Nutritional Demands: Creating eggs, sperm, and supporting pregnancy requires significant nutritional resources, highlighting why proper nutrition is fundamental to reproductive health.

COMMON STRUCTURAL CHALLENGES

While this book focuses primarily on functional approaches, it's important to recognize when structural issues may require medical intervention:

FEMALE STRUCTURAL ISSUES:
- Blocked fallopian tubes (requiring surgical repair, Clear Passage® therapy, or IVF)
- Uterine fibroids or polyps (may need removal)
- Endometriosis (addressed through both functional and medical approaches)
- Cervical scarring (may require surgical correction)

MALE STRUCTURAL ISSUES:
- Varicoceles (enlarged veins that may require surgical repair)
- Blocked vas deferens (may need surgical correction)
- Structural abnormalities (may require medical intervention)

The good news is that functional medicine approaches enhance the health of reproductive anatomy regardless of whether structural interventions are needed. By optimizing the environment in which these organs function, we give them the best possible chance to perform their remarkable roles in creating new life.

YOUR REPRODUCTIVE HOME RENOVATION

Now that you understand the basic layout and function of your reproductive home, you can better appreciate how the strategies in this book work to optimize each system. Just as a home renovation might upgrade the electrical system, improve the plumbing, and enhance the foundation, functional medicine approaches enhance hormonal signaling, improve circulation, and strengthen the overall environment supporting your reproductive anatomy.

In the sections that follow, we'll explore how hormones coordinate all these systems and how you can optimize that coordination for the best possible fertility outcomes. Remember, your reproductive anatomy has been designed for the remarkable purpose of creating life—our goal is simply to provide it with the optimal conditions to fulfill that purpose.

THE CLIMATE CONTROL SYSTEM: ENDOCRINE SYSTEM OVERVIEW

Just as a well-designed home requires sophisticated climate control to maintain comfort in every room and season, your body relies on an intricate endocrine system to regulate everything from metabolism to reproduction. This master 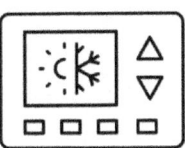 control system—your hormonal network—functions like a complex thermostat that continuously monitors conditions and makes precise adjustments to maintain optimal function.

The reproductive endocrine system, in particular, operates with remarkable precision, orchestrating the delicate dance between multiple glands and organs through an elegant system of feedback loops and chemical messengers. Understanding this system is essential for addressing any fertility challenges that arise.

In the next section, we'll explore the components of your reproductive hormone infrastructure, understanding both their individual roles and how they work together to create the optimal environment for conception and pregnancy.

CHAPTER 8

PRIMARY POWER SYSTEMS

ESSENTIAL FERTILITY INFRASTRUCTURE
POWER SUPPLY: ESTRADIOL

In our home renovation metaphor, estradiol—the primary form of estrogen during reproductive years—functions as the main power supply of your fertility system. Just as electricity energizes every aspect of a modern home, estradiol activates and powers numerous reproductive functions:

Primary Functions:
- **Follicular Development:** Stimulates growth of ovarian follicles housing eggs
- **Endometrial Building:** Triggers proliferation of uterine lining for potential implantation
- **Cervical Mucus Production:** Creates fertile-quality mucus that supports sperm survival

- **Libido Regulation:** Maintains sexual desire and function
- **Bone Density Maintenance:** Preserves skeletal strength for future pregnancy demands
- **Cognitive Function:** Supports brain health and emotional regulation

Production Sources:
- **Ovaries:** Primary source during reproductive years
- **Fat Tissue:** Secondary source that becomes more important with age
- **Adrenal Glands:** Minor but significant contribution
- **Placenta:** During pregnancy (producing estriol)

Regulation Mechanisms:
Estradiol levels rise and fall in a predictable pattern during a healthy menstrual cycle:
- **Follicular Phase:** Gradually increases, peaking just before ovulation
- **Ovulation:** Triggers the LH surge that leads to egg release
- **Luteal Phase:** Decreases after ovulation, then rises again midway through the luteal phase
- **Menstruation:** Drops to its lowest level during menstruation

Fertility Impact:
Proper estradiol function is crucial for fertility, affecting:
- Maturation of eggs within follicles
- Creation of sperm-friendly cervical mucus
- Development of a receptive endometrium
- Maintenance of proper bone density to support pregnancy

- Regulation of other reproductive hormones through feedback loops

Balance Considerations:
Like a home's electrical system, estradiol must be properly regulated:
- **Insufficient Estradiol:** Can lead to inadequate follicular development, thin endometrial lining, poor cervical mucus, and anovulation.
- **Excessive Estradiol:** May cause estrogen dominance, heavy periods, fibroids, endometriosis, and increased cancer risks in sensitive tissues (when poorly metabolized).

PROTECTIVE INSULATION: PROGESTERONE

If estradiol is the electrical system of your fertility home, progesterone serves as the protective insulation—ensuring safety, preventing short circuits, and enabling the power to flow properly without damaging the structure. Progesterone, meaning "pro-gestation," is literally the hormone that makes pregnancy possible.

Primary Functions:
- **Endometrial Preparation:** Transforms the uterine lining from proliferative to secretory phase
- **Implantation Support:** Creates a receptive environment for a fertilized egg
- **Pregnancy Maintenance:** Prevents uterine contractions and supports early pregnancy

- **Thermal Regulation:** Raises basal body temperature after ovulation
- **Mood Regulation:** Has calming, anti-anxiety effects on the nervous system
- **Immune Modulation:** Prevents rejection of the embryo (which contains "foreign" paternal DNA)

Production Sources:
- **Corpus Luteum:** The post-ovulatory follicle is the primary source
- **Adrenal Glands:** Produce small amounts
- **Placenta:** Takes over production around weeks 8–12 of pregnancy

Regulation Mechanisms:

Progesterone follows a distinct pattern during the menstrual cycle:
- **Follicular Phase:** Almost undetectable levels
- **Ovulation:** Begins rising after the egg is released
- **Luteal Phase:** Reaches peak levels 5–7 days after ovulation
- **Premenstrual:** Drops dramatically if no pregnancy occurs, triggering menstruation
- **Pregnancy:** Continues rising if conception occurs

Fertility Impact:

Progesterone's role in fertility is crucial:
- Prepares the endometrium for implantation
- Maintains the uterine lining during early pregnancy
- Prevents premature uterine contractions that could disrupt implantation

- Supports the immunological changes needed to accept the embryo
- Signals to the hypothalamus to prevent further ovulation during pregnancy

Balance Considerations:
Just as improper insulation can cause electrical hazards or energy inefficiency:
- **Insufficient Progesterone:** Can cause luteal phase defects, implantation failure, early miscarriage, PMS, anxiety, and sleep disturbances.
- **Excessive Progesterone:** Rarely occurs naturally but can cause excessive sedation, bloating, and breast tenderness when supplemented inappropriately.

STRUCTURAL SUPPORT: TESTOSTERONE, DHEA, AND DHT

In our home renovation metaphor, androgens like testosterone, DHEA, and DHT function as the structural support system—the beams, joists, and framework that provide strength and form to the entire fertility structure. While often considered "male" hormones, these androgens play essential roles in female fertility as well.

TESTOSTERONE
Primary Functions:
- **Ovarian Stimulation:** Supports follicular development and ovulation
- **Libido Maintenance:** Drives sexual desire in both men and women

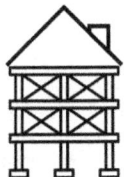

Primary Power Systems 85

- **Energy Production:** Contributes to overall vitality and muscle strength
- **Bone Density:** Maintains skeletal integrity
- **Cognitive Function:** Supports mental clarity, drive, and motivation
- **Production Sources:**
- **Women:** Ovaries and adrenal glands (producing about 1/10th of male levels)
- **Men:** Primarily testes (95%), with small amounts from adrenal glands

DHEA (DEHYDROEPIANDROSTERONE)

Primary Functions:

- **Hormone Precursor:** Serves as building block for both testosterone and estrogen
- **Immune Support:** Enhances immune system function
- **Stress Resilience:** Provides counterbalance to cortisol effects
- **Cognitive Protection:** Supports brain health and function

Production Sources:

- Primarily produced in the adrenal glands
- Small amounts produced in the ovaries
- Peaks in early adulthood and gradually declines with age

DHT (DIHYDROTESTOSTERONE)

Primary Functions:

- **Secondary Sexual Characteristics:** Drives male-pattern hair growth
- **Skin Oil Production:** Affects sebaceous gland activity
- **Hair Follicle Regulation:** Influences scalp hair patterns

Production Sources:
- Converted from testosterone in tissue via the enzyme 5-alpha reductase
- Primarily important in male development but impacts women as well

Fertility Impact:
The role of androgens in fertility includes:
- Supporting early follicular development in women
- Maintaining healthy libido for regular intercourse
- Providing the energy reserves needed for reproduction
- In men, driving sperm production and sexual function
- Balancing with estrogen for optimal reproductive function

Balance Considerations:
Like structural elements in a home, these hormones must be properly proportioned:
- **Insufficient Androgens:** Can lead to fatigue, low libido, poor follicular development, decreased muscle mass, and mood changes.
- **Excessive Androgens in Women:** May cause PCOS, hirsutism, hair loss, acne, irregular cycles, and infertility.
- **Excessive DHT in Men:** Can contribute to male pattern baldness and prostate issues.

CHAPTER 9

SUPPORT AND ENVIRONMENTAL SYSTEMS

BACKUP SYSTEMS: PREGNENOLONE AND CORTISOL

In our home renovation metaphor, pregnenolone and cortisol function as the backup generator and emergency response systems. When stress or high demand threatens your home's normal operations, these systems activate to ensure essential functions continue. Similarly, these hormones respond to stress and help prioritize resources during challenging times.

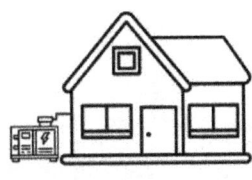

PREGNENOLONE
Primary Functions:
- **Master Hormone Precursor:** Serves as the primary building block for nearly all steroid hormones
- **Neurological Protection:** Supports brain function and memory

- **Stress Adaptation:** Provides raw material for stress response hormones when needed
- **Mood Regulation:** Influences GABA and dopamine systems in the brain

Production Sources:
- Primarily manufactured in the adrenal glands
- Also produced in smaller amounts in the brain, liver, skin, and gonads
- Derived from cholesterol through a multi-step conversion process

Fertility Impact:
- Ensures adequate raw materials for producing reproductive hormones
- Supports cognitive and emotional health necessary for fertility
- Enables appropriate stress response without depleting reproductive function
- Maintains hormonal reserve capacity for pregnancy demands

CORTISOL
Primary Functions:
- **Stress Response Coordination:** Primary hormone of the "fight or flight" response
- **Energy Mobilization:** Raises blood sugar to provide fuel during stress
- **Immune Regulation:** Modulates inflammation and immune activity
- **Circadian Rhythm:** Helps maintain proper sleep-wake cycles

- **Blood Pressure Regulation:** Increases blood pressure during stress response

Production Sources:
- Produced by the adrenal cortex
- Release is triggered by ACTH from the pituitary gland
- Follows a natural daily rhythm (highest in morning, lowest at night)

Fertility Impact:
- When balanced, helps the body respond appropriately to stress without compromising reproduction
- When chronically elevated, can "steal" pregnenolone from reproductive hormone pathways (pregnenolone steal)
- Affects thyroid function, which indirectly impacts fertility
- Influences insulin sensitivity and metabolic health
- Regulates immune function, which affects implantation and pregnancy maintenance

Balance Considerations:
Just as backup systems must be properly calibrated:
- **Insufficient Pregnenolone:** Can limit production of all downstream hormones, leading to fatigue, poor stress tolerance, and reduced fertility.
- **Insufficient Cortisol:** May cause fatigue, hypoglycemia, low blood pressure, poor stress tolerance, and inflammatory issues.
- **Excessive Cortisol:** Can suppress reproductive function, disrupt sleep, reduce immune function, decrease bone density, and contribute to insulin resistance.

- **Dysregulated Cortisol Rhythm:** May disrupt sleep-wake cycles, impair recovery, and affect reproductive hormone pulsatility.

PLUMBING SYSTEMS: PROLACTIN

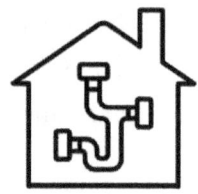

In our home renovation metaphor, prolactin functions like the plumbing system—essential for nurturing new life once it arrives, but potentially disruptive if activated at the wrong time or in excessive amounts. Just as water is vital for a home but damaging if pipes leak where they shouldn't, prolactin must be precisely regulated for optimal fertility.

Primary Functions:
- **Milk Production:** Stimulates mammary glands to produce breast milk
- **Immune Support:** Enhances immune system function
- **Reproductive Regulation:** Influences ovulation and luteal function
- **Osmoregulation:** Helps maintain water and electrolyte balance
- **Metabolism:** Affects insulin sensitivity and fat storage

Production Sources:
- Primarily produced by the anterior pituitary gland
- Small amounts also produced in the brain, immune cells, uterus, and mammary glands
- Production increases dramatically during pregnancy and breastfeeding

Regulation Mechanisms:
- **Dopamine:** Primary inhibitory control (higher dopamine = lower prolactin)
- **Estrogen:** Stimulates prolactin production
- **Stress Hormones:** Acute stress can temporarily increase prolactin
- **Sleep:** Levels naturally rise during sleep, peaking in the early morning
- **Physical Stimulation:** Breast/nipple stimulation increases production
- **TRH:** Thyroid-releasing hormone also stimulates prolactin

Fertility Impact:
Prolactin's relationship with fertility is complex:
- **Normal Levels:** Support corpus luteum function and progesterone production
- **Elevated Levels:** Can suppress gonadotropin-releasing hormone (GnRH) pulsatility, inhibiting ovulation and menstruation
- **Postpartum:** High levels during breastfeeding often prevent ovulation (natural child spacing)
- **Emotional Component:** Influences nurturing behaviors and maternal bonding

Balance Considerations:
Like plumbing in a home, prolactin must function properly at the right times:
- **Insufficient Prolactin:** Rarely a concern for fertility, but causes inability to produce breast milk after childbirth.

- **Elevated Prolactin (Hyperprolactinemia):** Can cause irregular or absent periods, infertility, galactorrhea (inappropriate milk production), reduced libido, and sometimes vision changes if caused by a pituitary tumor (prolactinoma).
- **Common Causes of Elevation:** Stress, certain medications (especially antipsychotics), pituitary tumors, hypothyroidism, and excessive breast stimulation.

ENVIRONMENTAL CONTROLS: THYROID HORMONES

In our home renovation metaphor, thyroid hormones function as the environmental control system—regulating metabolism, energy use, and temperature throughout the entire structure. Like a sophisticated HVAC 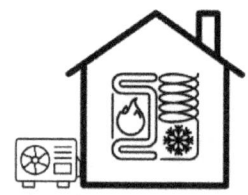 system that ensures every room maintains optimal conditions, thyroid hormones influence virtually every cell in your body, creating the perfect metabolic environment for fertility and reproduction.

PRIMARY THYROID HORMONES:

T4 (Thyroxine):
- The primary hormone secreted by the thyroid gland
- Acts mainly as a prohormone that converts to the more active T3
- Has a longer half-life, providing stable baseline levels

T3 (Triiodothyronine):
- The more metabolically active form
- Primarily created through conversion from T4 in tissues
- Directly interacts with nuclear receptors to affect genetic expression
- Gas pedal on all things thyroid

Reverse T3 (rT3):
- An inactive form produced during stress or illness
- Acts as a metabolic pause during challenging times
- Brake pedal on all things thyroid
- Can block receptor sites for active T3

Primary Functions:
- **Metabolic Regulation:** Controls the rate at which cells convert nutrients to energy
- **Temperature Regulation:** Maintains proper body temperature
- **Protein Synthesis:** Influences production of enzymes and structural proteins
- **Brain Development:** Critical for neurological development and function
- **Cardiovascular Regulation:** Affects heart rate and cardiac output
- **Muscle Control:** Influences muscle contraction and relaxation
- **Digestive Function:** Regulates digestive secretions and motility
- **Bone Metabolism:** Influences bone turnover and density

Production and Regulation:
- **Hypothalamic-Pituitary-Thyroid (HPT) Axis:**
    - Hypothalamus produces TRH (Thyrotropin-Releasing Hormone)
    - TRH stimulates pituitary to release TSH (Thyroid-Stimulating Hormone)
    - TSH triggers thyroid gland to produce T4 and some T3
    - T4 converts to active T3 in peripheral tissues (liver, kidneys, muscles)
    - Proper function requires adequate iodine, tyrosine, selenium, zinc, magnesium, and other nutrients

Fertility Impact:
Thyroid function profoundly affects fertility in numerous ways:
- **Ovulation:** Regulates menstrual cycle regularity and ovulation
- **Egg Quality:** Influences follicular development and maturation
- **Progesterone Production:** Affects luteal phase adequacy
- **Estrogen Balance:** Impacts estrogen metabolism and clearance
- **Implantation:** Affects endometrial receptivity
- **Pregnancy Maintenance:** Critical for early embryonic development
- **Male Fertility:** Influences sperm production, morphology, and motility
- **Libido:** Affects sexual desire in both men and women
- **Metabolic Health:** Influences insulin sensitivity and weight management

Balance Considerations:

Like environmental controls in a home, thyroid function must be precisely balanced:

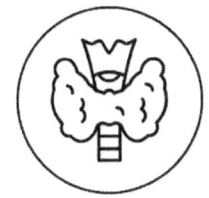

- **Hypothyroidism (Insufficient):** Can cause menstrual irregularities, anovulation, luteal phase defects, recurrent miscarriage, fatigue, cold intolerance, constipation, dry skin, hair loss, and weight gain resistant to diet and exercise.
- **Hyperthyroidism (Excessive):** May lead to irregular periods, shorter cycles, reduced menstrual flow, anxiety, heart palpitations, heat intolerance, weight loss despite increased appetite, and insomnia.
- **Subclinical Thyroid Dysfunction:** Even mild imbalances within "normal" laboratory ranges can impact fertility, particularly if thyroid peroxidase antibodies (TPOABs) are present (Hashimoto's thyroiditis).
- **Autoimmune Thyroid Disease:** Associated with other reproductive autoimmune conditions and increased risk of pregnancy complications.
- **Optimal Fertility Ranges:** For conception and pregnancy, many functional medicine practitioners target TSH between 1.0–2.5 mIU/L, free T3 in the upper half of the reference range, and free T4 in the mid to upper portion of the reference range if tolerated by the patient.

CHAPTER 10

SYSTEM INTEGRATION—MONTHLY PATTERNS AND ASSESSMENT

KEY HORMONE FUNCTIONS DURING CYCLE
Estradiol (Primary Estrogen)
- Peak Times: Day 12–14 (ovulation), Day 20–22 (luteal phase secondary peak)
- Functions: Builds uterine lining, stimulates cervical mucus production, supports follicle development
- Fertility Signs: Increasing cervical mucus quality, improved mood and energy

Progesterone
- Peak Time: Days 19–22 (mid-luteal phase)
- Functions: Maintains uterine lining, supports implantation, raises body temperature
- Fertility Signs: Temperature rise after ovulation, dry cervical mucus, premenstrual symptoms if excessive

MENSTRUAL CYCLE HORMONE PATTERNS

The Monthly Symphony: "How Your Hormones Dance Together"

VISUAL HORMONE PATTERN CHART (28-DAY CYCLE)

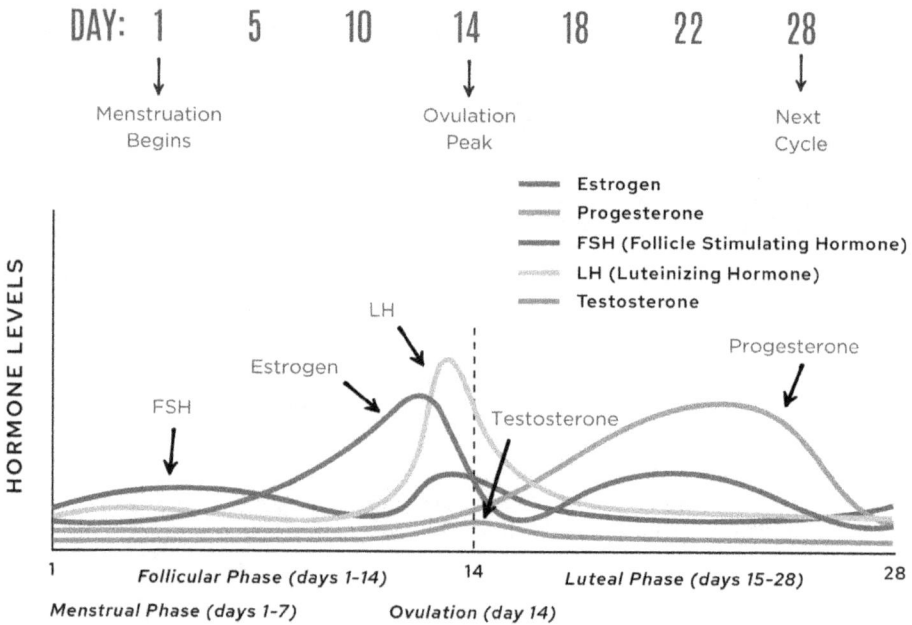

DETAILED HORMONE TIMELINE TABLE

Cycle Phase	Days	Dominant Hormones	Hormone Levels	What's Happening
Menstrual Phase	1–5	Low across all hormones	Estrogen: LOW Progesterone: LOW FSH: Beginning to rise LH: LOW	-Uterine lining sheds -New follicles begin developing -Energy typically lowest
Follicular Phase	1–13	FSH rising, Estrogen climbing	FSH: HIGH (days 1–7) Estrogen: RISING steadily Progesterone: LOW LH: LOW Testosterone: Gradual rise	-Follicles mature -Dominant follicle selected -Uterine lining begins rebuilding -Energy increasing
Ovulatory Phase	12–16	LH surge, Estrogen peak	LH: MASSIVE SURGE (24–48 hrs) Estrogen: PEAK then sharp drop FSH: Secondary surge Testosterone: PEAK Progesterone: Beginning to rise	-Egg released from follicle -Peak fertility window -Highest energy and libido -BBT begins to rise
Luteal Phase	15–28	Progesterone dominant	Progesterone: PEAK (days 19–22) Estrogen: Moderate rise then fall LH: LOW FSH: LOW Testosterone: Declining	-Corpus luteum maintains lining -If no pregnancy: hormone crash -PMS symptoms may appear -Energy stabilizing then declining

Luteinizing Hormone (LH)
- Peak Time: Days 12–14 (ovulation surge lasting 24–48 hours)
- Functions: Triggers ovulation, stimulates corpus luteum formation
- Fertility Signs: Detected by ovulation predictor kits, peak fertility window

Follicle Stimulating Hormone (FSH)
- Peak Times: Days 1–7 (early follicular), Day 13–14 (ovulation), Days 26–28 (late luteal)
- Functions: Stimulates follicle growth, supports egg maturation
- Fertility Signs: Early cycle energy, preparation for next cycle

Testosterone
- Peak Time: Days 10–14 (around ovulation)
- Functions: Supports libido, contributes to follicle development, enhances energy
- Fertility Signs: Increased sex drive, assertiveness, physical strength

OPTIMAL TIMING FOR FERTILITY ACTIVITIES

Activity	Best Timing	Hormone Rationale
Hormone Testing	Day 3: FSH, LH, Estradiol Day 21: Progesterone	Day 3: Baseline levels Day 21: Peak progesterone confirms ovulation
Intense Exercise	Days 5-13	Rising estrogen supports energy; avoid during luteal phase when progesterone dominates
Social Activities	Days 8-16	Rising estrogen and testosterone enhance mood and social energy
Conception Attempts	Days 12-16	LH surge indicates impending ovulation; peak estrogen creates optimal cervical mucus
Stress Management Focus	Days 19-28	High progesterone can amplify stress responses; PMS symptoms emerge

WHAT OPTIMAL PATTERNS LOOK LIKE

Healthy Cycle Indicators:

- Cycle length: 26–35 days consistently
- Temperature rise: 0.2–0.4°F sustained for 12–14 days after ovulation
- Cervical mucus: Clear, stretchy "egg white" quality around ovulation
- Energy patterns: Increasing through follicular phase, peak at ovulation, stable in luteal phase
- Minimal PMS: Mild symptoms if any in the 2–3 days before menstruation

Concerning Patterns:
- Cycles shorter than 21 days or longer than 35 days
- No temperature rise (may indicate anovulation)
- Luteal phase shorter than 10 days
- Severe PMS lasting more than 3–4 days
- No fertile cervical mucus around expected ovulation

Clinical Pearl for Practitioners
Understanding these hormone patterns allows for precise timing of interventions:
- Seed cycling protocols can be aligned with natural hormone phases
- Supplement timing can be optimized (e.g., progesterone support in luteal phase)
- Testing schedules provide maximum diagnostic information
- Lifestyle recommendations can be cycle-specific for better compliance and results

This hormone choreography represents one of nature's most elegant systems—when functioning optimally, it creates the perfect conditions for new life while maintaining overall health and vitality.

THE INTEGRATION OF HORMONAL SYSTEMS

The true marvel of your reproductive endocrine system lies not just in the individual components but in how they work together in perfect coordination. Like a well-designed home where the electrical, plumbing, HVAC, and structural systems are integrated into a seamless whole, your hormonal systems must function in harmony.

Key Integration Points:
1. **The Hypothalamic-Pituitary-Ovarian Axis**
    - The command center (hypothalamus) monitors conditions throughout the body
    - The control relay (pituitary) sends specific signals to the reproductive organs
    - The end organs (ovaries/testes) both respond to signals and provide feedback

2. **The Adrenal-Gonadal Connection**
    - Stress response systems communicate constantly with reproductive systems
    - Both systems draw from the same precursor hormones (pregnenolone)
    - Resource allocation shifts based on perceived priorities (survival vs. reproduction)

3. **The Thyroid-Reproductive Relationship**
    - Thyroid function affects reproductive hormone production and metabolism
    - Reproductive hormones influence thyroid hormone binding and activity
    - Both systems are sensitive to nutritional status and environmental factors

4. **The Insulin-Hormone Balance**
    - Insulin sensitivity affects ovarian hormone production (especially in PCOS)

- Sex hormones influence fat distribution and insulin response
- Blood sugar stability impacts hormone balance and egg quality

5. **The Gut-Hormone Connection**
   - Gut microbiome influences estrogen recycling and detoxification
   - Digestive health affects hormone absorption and nutrient availability
   - Inflammation in the gut can trigger systemic inflammation affecting reproduction

Understanding these integration points helps explain why *isolated* hormone treatments often fail to resolve fertility challenges. Just as fixing a home's electrical system won't solve a problem with the foundation, *addressing a single hormone without considering the entire system may not produce lasting results.*

In functional medicine, we recognize that creating optimal hormonal balance requires a comprehensive approach—ensuring that each system is working properly while also optimizing the communication and coordination between systems.

HORMONE TESTING: INSPECTING YOUR SYSTEMS

Just as a home inspector uses specialized tools and methods to evaluate a property's condition, we can assess hormonal health through various testing methods. Each approach has strengths and limitations, and often a combination provides the most complete picture.

As I first shared in *Your Longevity Blueprint*, just as human fingerprints are detailed, unique markers of human identity, so are your fertility test results. No two women have identical hormone patterns or eggs, and no two men have identical sperm parameters. Your comprehensive testing creates a unique "fertility fingerprint" that reveals the specific imbalances, deficiencies, and dysfunction patterns affecting your reproductive health.

These detailed results allow your healthcare provider to personalize a fertility renovation plan specifically for your body's needs, rather than applying generic protocols that may not address your individual challenges. **Your fertility fingerprint becomes the blueprint for your personalized path to parenthood.**

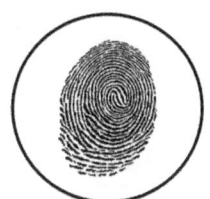

COMMON HORMONE TESTING METHODS:

1. **Serum (Blood) Testing:**
    - Measures hormones circulating in bloodstream
    - Provides point-in-time snapshot of hormone levels
    - Most conventional medical testing uses this method
    - Best for: Thyroid hormones, prolactin, estradiol (on specific cycle days), LH, FSH

2. **Saliva Testing:**
    - Measures free (unbound) hormone that is bioavailable to tissues
    - Less invasive than blood testing
    - Allows for multiple samples throughout day or month
    - Best for: Cortisol rhythm assessment, progesterone/estrogen patterns across cycle

3. **Urine Testing:**
   - Measures metabolites and breakdown products
   - Reveals how hormones are being processed
   - DUTCH (Dried Urine Test for Comprehensive Hormones) provides detailed metabolite information
   - Best for: Estrogen metabolism pathways, cortisol metabolites, androgen metabolism

Functional Challenges:
   - Evaluates hormone response to specific stimuli
   - Examples include thyrotropin-releasing hormone (TRH) stimulation test, adrenocorticotropic hormone (ACTH) challenge, glucose tolerance test
   - Best for: Assessing hormone reserve capacity and feedback mechanisms

TIMING CONSIDERATIONS:

For women, hormone testing must consider cycle timing:
- **Follicular Phase Testing (Days 2–4):** FSH, LH, estradiol for ovarian reserve
- **Mid-Cycle (Days 12–16):** Estradiol, LH for ovulation assessment
- **Luteal Phase (Days 19–22):** Progesterone for ovulation confirmation and luteal adequacy
- **Full-Cycle Mapping:** Multiple samples throughout month for comprehensive assessment

INTERPRETATION PRINCIPLES:

When evaluating hormone test results, remember:

1. **Optimal vs. Normal Ranges:** Laboratory "normal" ranges often reflect statistical norms rather than optimal fertility levels.
2. **Ratios Matter:** The relationship between hormones (e.g., estrogen/progesterone ratio) can be more important than absolute values.
3. **Patterns Over Points:** A single measurement rarely tells the complete story—trends and patterns provide more insight.
4. **Individual Variation:** Each person has a unique "optimal" set point that may differ from population averages.
5. **Symptom Correlation:** Test results should be interpreted in context of clinical symptoms and fertility outcomes.

In the next section, we'll explore how these hormonal systems can malfunction, creating the structural challenges that impact fertility, and how both conventional and functional approaches address these issues.

SECTION IV

STRUCTURAL CHALLENGES—DIAGNOSING AND ADDRESSING FERTILITY OBSTACLES

CHAPTER 11

COMMON STRUCTURAL ISSUES

Just as a house needs solid foundations, proper wiring, and functioning plumbing to be livable, your body requires certain structural elements to be in optimal condition for fertility. When these systems malfunction, conception becomes more challenging. In this and subsequent chapters, we'll explore common structural fertility challenges using our home renovation metaphor, helping you understand both conventional "quick fixes" and more comprehensive functional medicine approaches.

ENDOMETRIOSIS: OVERGROWN INTERIOR WALLS

Imagine your body as a home where the interior wall material (endometrial tissue) has begun growing outside its designated areas. This is endometriosis—tissue similar to your uterine lining appearing on your ovaries, fallopian tubes, and pelvic tissues. Just as misplaced building materials would disrupt a home's functionality, this misplaced tissue creates inflammation, pain, and potential fertility challenges.

Endometriosis impacts roughly 10% of reproductive-age women, though most don't receive a diagnosis until their thirties or forties. The numbers become even more striking when we look at women struggling with infertility—up to 50% may have endometriosis. Perhaps most telling is that approximately 70% of women dealing with chronic pelvic pain have this condition, often after years of being told their pain is "normal" or psychological.

INSPECTION METHODS: SYMPTOMS AND DIAGNOSIS
Primary Warning Signs:
- Severe menstrual cramps that exceed typical discomfort
- Pain during intercourse
- Pain with bowel movements or urination during menstrual periods
- Excessive bleeding during or between periods
- Infertility

Much like a home inspector might need to look behind walls to identify problems, endometriosis often requires a surgical procedure called laparoscopy for definitive diagnosis. Your doctor may first use:

- Detailed symptom history
- Pelvic examinations
- Ultrasound imaging
- MRI scanning

However, laparoscopy—where a surgeon inserts a slender viewing instrument through a small abdominal incision—remains the gold standard for diagnosis, allowing visual confirmation of endometrial tissue growing where it shouldn't be.

MY PERSONAL JOURNEY WITH ENDOMETRIOSIS

My own experience with endometriosis underscores the importance of proper diagnosis and treatment. Despite having textbook symptoms—extremely painful, heavy periods that had become somewhat manageable through anti-inflammatory nutrition, progesterone support, and supplements like turmeric, magnesium, and fish oil—I repeatedly received normal results on hormone panels and ultrasounds showing regular ovulation.

After multiple failed IUIs despite seemingly "perfect" hormone levels, I suspected endometriosis might be the hidden factor in my fertility struggles. Local friends who had undergone standard surgical approaches had experienced quick recurrence without achieving pregnancy, so I researched specialists who used advanced techniques with lower recurrence rates. Thankfully, my primary care physician, Dr. Monica Minjeur, was of great help. She led me to the Pope Paul Institute in Omaha, Nebraska, where exploratory surgery confirmed my suspicions: I had stage 4 endometriosis. The diagnosis was both validating and devastating. While I can look back now with gratitude for this discovery, the journey was challenging. Following surgery, complications with our trip home turned a four-hour drive into an eight-hour ordeal, complete with a flat tire that left me waiting on the interstate, nauseous, in pain, and worried my incisions were compromising. Soaked in sweat in the hot Iowa summer, needless to say I was discouraged—but I had answers.

I later returned for a successful robotic surgery using their specialized non-scarring technique, which reduced recurrence rates from over 50% to approximately 7%. This experience taught me firsthand that standard testing often misses significant structural issues like endometriosis and that seeking specialized care can make the difference between continued struggling and finding real answers.

CONVENTIONAL PATCHES VS. FUNCTIONAL REBUILDING APPROACHES
CONVENTIONAL APPROACHES (THE QUICK FIX):

The conventional medical approach to endometriosis often resembles applying temporary patches to leaking walls:

1. **Pain Management:** NSAIDs like ibuprofen to reduce inflammation and pain
2. **Hormonal Treatments:** Birth control pills, patches, or hormonal IUDs to suppress menstruation and reduce painful symptoms
3. **GnRH therapy:** Medications that block reproductive hormones, inducing a temporary menopausal state
4. **Surgical Intervention:** Laparoscopic surgery to remove endometrial growths, which may provide temporary relief but often sees the tissue return within years

These approaches primarily focus on symptom management rather than addressing root causes, similar to patching a leaking wall without investigating why the water is coming in.

FUNCTIONAL REBUILDING APPROACHES (THE COMPREHENSIVE RENOVATION):

Functional medicine approaches endometriosis as a full-scale renovation project, addressing the underlying causes of tissue overgrowth:

1. **Natural Pain Management Strategies:** Castor oil packs have been used therapeutically for centuries and may offer significant benefits for women with endometriosis. When applied topically over the lower abdomen and pelvis, castor oil's ricinoleic acid penetrates deeply into tissues, promoting lymphatic drainage and reducing inflammation—both crucial

for managing endometriosis symptoms. Many women report decreased pelvic pain, reduced menstrual cramping, and improved cycle regularity after consistent use. The application process itself—lying still with heat for 45–60 minutes—also activates the parasympathetic nervous system, promoting relaxation and stress reduction, which further supports hormonal balance. For optimal results, apply castor oil packs 3–4 times weekly during the luteal phase of your cycle (after ovulation until menstruation begins), avoiding use during menstruation and the first half of your cycle if you're actively trying to conceive. Use only hexane-free castor oil stored in glass bottles.

2. **Anti-Inflammatory Nutrition:**
    - Eliminating inflammatory foods (gluten, dairy, processed foods, sugar)
    - Emphasizing omega-3-rich foods (wild-caught fish, walnuts, flaxseeds)
    - Increasing antioxidant intake through colorful vegetables and fruits
    - Supporting liver detoxification with cruciferous vegetables

3. **Hormone Balancing:**
    - Reducing xenoestrogens from plastics, conventional beauty products, and household cleaners
    - Supporting healthy estrogen metabolism through specific nutrients (DIM, calcium d-glucarate)
    - Using targeted supplements like magnesium, vitamin E, and B vitamins

4. **Gut Health Restoration:**
    - Healing intestinal permeability, which contributes to inflammation
    - Balancing the microbiome with probiotics and prebiotic foods
    - Identifying and addressing food sensitivities

THE CRITICAL GUT-UTERUS CONNECTION:

The connection between gut health and endometriosis cannot be overstated. As obstetrician-gynecologist Dr. Tabatha Barber shared with me during an interview on my Your Longevity Blueprint podcast, surgeons literally have to move the bowels out of the way when operating in the pelvic cavity—the intestines are in direct physical contact with the uterus. This anatomical reality means inflammation in your digestive tract directly affects your reproductive organs.

Think of it this way: when your gut is inflamed, it's like having a smoldering fire right next to the walls of your reproductive home. That heat and inflammatory damage inevitably spread to adjacent structures. Conversely, when you reduce gut inflammation, you're essentially creating a fire break that protects your reproductive organs.

This connection was hugely important in my own fertility journey. I had been gluten-free for years while trying to conceive my first son, which helped manage some symptoms. However, my comprehensive food sensitivity testing also revealed significant reactions to dairy products. It was exactly one year after eliminating dairy completely from my diet that I finally conceived. This timing wasn't coincidental—reducing the inflammatory burden in my digestive tract, which sits directly against the reproductive organs, created a more hospitable environment for conception. The gut-uterine connection was a crucial piece of my fertility puzzle.

Research increasingly supports this relationship, showing that women with endometriosis have higher rates of gut dysbiosis, food sensitivities, and intestinal permeability compared to women without the condition. By addressing these gut issues, you're not just improving digestive function—you're directly influencing the environment where endometriosis develops and potentially removing a significant barrier to fertility.

5. Stress Reduction Protocols:
- o Implementing mindfulness practices
- o Prioritizing adequate sleep
- o Incorporating gentle movement like yoga or walking

6. Environmental Toxin Reduction:
- o Switching to natural cleaning products
- o Using clean beauty products
- o Filtering water and air

Just as a quality renovation addresses the root causes of structural problems rather than simply covering them up, this comprehensive approach seeks to create an environment where endometriosis is less likely to progress, potentially restoring fertility without the side effects associated with conventional treatments.

> **Success Story:** Sarah struggled with endometriosis for eight years, experiencing debilitating pain and trying unsuccessfully to conceive. After two laparoscopic surgeries provided only temporary relief, she adopted a functional medicine approach. Six months of anti-inflammatory nutrition, hormone-balancing supplements, low-dose naltrexone (LDN), and stress-reduction techniques not only reduced her pain significantly but also resulted in a natural pregnancy after years of trying.

PCOS: ELECTRICAL SYSTEM IRREGULARITIES

If your reproductive system were a house, polycystic ovary syndrome (PCOS) would be like electrical system irregularities—the lights flicker, some circuits overload while others don't receive enough power, and the whole system becomes unreliable. In PCOS, your hormonal circuitry  misfires: insulin levels surge, testosterone increases, and the delicate balance needed for regular ovulation becomes disrupted.

While PCOS affects 6–20% of reproductive-age women, the staggering reality is that approximately 70% remain undiagnosed. This diagnostic gap means countless women are told their fertility struggles are "unexplained" or that they simply need to "lose weight and try harder," when in fact they have a specific hormonal condition that can be effectively addressed through functional medicine approaches.

CIRCUIT TESTING: SYMPTOMS AND DIAGNOSIS

Warning Indicators:

Just as flickering lights and tripped breakers signal electrical problems, PCOS has its own warning signs:

- **Irregular or Absent Menstrual Cycles:** The most common circuit malfunction, indicating ovulation may not be occurring regularly
- **Excess Androgens:** Manifesting as unwanted hair growth (hirsutism), acne, or male-pattern baldness
- **Polycystic Ovaries:** Multiple small follicles on the ovaries that appear like a string of pearls on ultrasound
- **Weight Challenges:** Particularly around the midsection, affecting approximately 80% of women with PCOS
- **Skin Tags and Darkened Skin Patches:** Often around the neck, armpits, or under breasts (acanthosis nigricans)
- **Fertility Difficulties:** Trouble conceiving due to irregular ovulation

Diagnostic Circuit Testing:

Like a thorough electrical inspection, diagnosing PCOS typically involves multiple tests:

1. **Medical History Review:** Your doctor will discuss your menstrual patterns, weight changes, and other symptoms
2. **Physical Examination:** Assessment of blood pressure, BMI, waist circumference, skin changes, and hair growth patterns
3. **Transvaginal Ultrasound:** To examine ovarian follicles and uterine lining—similar to inspecting your electrical panel and wiring

4. **Blood Tests:** The comprehensive circuit analysis:
   - Hormone levels (testosterone, DHEA-S, androstenedione, DHT)
   - Glucose tolerance and insulin levels
   - Cholesterol and triglyceride measurements
   - Thyroid function tests
   - Prolactin levels

According to the Rotterdam criteria, you need at least two of these three conditions for diagnosis:

- Irregular or absent menstrual cycles
- Signs of excess androgens (either physical symptoms or blood test results)
- Polycystic ovaries on ultrasound

STANDARD REPAIRS VS. COMPLETE REWIRING SOLUTIONS
Standard Repairs (Conventional Approach):

Conventional PCOS treatment resembles applying partial fixes to an electrical system without addressing the underlying wiring issues:

1. **Birth Control Pills:** Act like circuit stabilizers to regulate periods and reduce androgen levels, but don't address the root cause of hormone imbalance
2. **Metformin:** Functions as a power regulator to improve insulin sensitivity, particularly effective for women with insulin resistance or prediabetes
3. **Clomid or Letrozole:** Serve as temporary circuit boosters to induce ovulation when trying to conceive
4. **Spironolactone or Anti-Androgens:** Work as targeted circuit reducers to decrease testosterone effects for acne and

hair growth (Note: These shouldn't be taken when you are actively trying to conceive)
5. **Symptom-Specific Treatments:** Treatments like laser hair removal, acne medications, or weight-loss medications that address individual symptoms rather than the underlying condition

While these approaches may provide relief and improve fertility in the short term, they rarely address the fundamental electrical system malfunctions driving PCOS.

Complete Rewiring Solutions (Functional Approach):
The functional medicine approach to PCOS is like rewiring your entire electrical system for optimal performance:

1. **Insulin Regulation:** The master circuit breaker
    - Low-glycemic diet minimizing processed carbs and sugars
    - Strategic meal timing and composition (protein + fiber with each meal)
    - Key supplements: inositol (particularly myo-inositol and D-chiro-inositol in a 40:1 ratio), berberine, chromium, and alpha-lipoic acid
    - Intermittent fasting protocols customized for hormone balance

2. **Anti-Inflammatory Lifestyle:** Reducing system-wide circuit overloading
    - Identifying and eliminating inflammatory foods including gluten, dairy, processed oils (Note: Your

functional medicine provider can test you to see what foods specifically you are sensitive to)
- Emphasizing omega-3-rich foods and antioxidants
- Regular, appropriate exercise with emphasis on strength training and high-intensity interval training (HIIT)
- Stress management through mindfulness, adequate sleep, and boundary setting

3. **Gut Microbiome Restoration:** Optimizing the control center
   - Probiotic-rich foods and supplements
   - Prebiotic fiber to feed beneficial bacteria
   - Identifying and removing gut irritants
   - Addressing intestinal permeability (leaky gut)

4. **Hormone Detoxification Support:** Ensuring proper circuit clearing
   - Supporting liver function with cruciferous vegetables, milk thistle, and glutathione precursors
   - Reducing environmental toxin exposure
   - Ensuring regular bowel movements
   - Optimizing nutrient cofactors for detoxification pathways

5. **Adrenal Support:** Balancing the backup power system
   - Adaptogenic herbs like ashwagandha and rhodiola
   - Vitamin C and B-complex supplementation
   - Cortisol rhythm normalization through morning light exposure and evening blue light reduction
   - Stress reduction techniques and appropriate exercise intensity

> **Success Story:** Jennifer had struggled with PCOS for over a decade, with irregular periods occurring only 3-4 times per year, persistent acne, and difficulty maintaining her weight despite constant dieting. After multiple doctors offered only birth control pills and weight loss advice, she worked with a functional medicine practitioner who identified significant insulin resistance and inflammation. Through a personalized protocol focusing on blood sugar regulation, specific supplements including inositol and NAC, and anti-inflammatory nutrition, Jennifer experienced regular monthly cycles for the first time in her adult life. Three months later, she was surprised to discover she was pregnant naturally after years of believing she would need fertility treatments.

This is not a unique case. I've seen several PCOS patients in my clinic who were told they would never conceive. I disagreed. They had never been offered a functional medicine approach. Through food-sensitivity testing, the use of diet and lifestyle changes, and supplements to correct insulin resistance and boost progesterone, we assisted them in achieving their goals more easily than they anticipated. One patient in particular, a long-time patient of mine who had a strong family history of diabetes and personal history of PCOS, became very serious about her ability to conceive, ate very clean, and incorporated HIIT training, heavy detox programs, and antiandrogenic herbs, and she was able to conceive without medications. She delivered her healthy baby girl shortly after I delivered Michael!

ADVANCED ELECTRICAL SYSTEM SUPPORT: PHARMACEUTICAL OPTIONS

Metformin and GLP-1 Agonists: Pharmaceutical Support for Insulin Resistance and Fertility

While the foundation of addressing insulin resistance should always begin with nutrition and lifestyle modifications, some individuals benefit from pharmaceutical support to restore proper glucose metabolism and enhance fertility outcomes. In our home renovation metaphor, these medications function like specialized power tools that can accomplish tasks more efficiently than manual methods alone—they're not replacements for good technique, but they can accelerate and enhance results when used appropriately.

METFORMIN: THE TIME-TESTED INSULIN SENSITIZER

Metformin, originally derived from the French lilac plant, has been used for diabetes management for decades but has shown remarkable benefits for fertility, particularly in women with PCOS and insulin resistance.

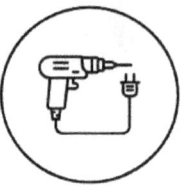

Mechanisms of Action for Fertility:
- Improved Insulin Sensitivity: Reduces insulin resistance, allowing cells to respond better to insulin signals
- Reduced Androgen Production: Lower insulin levels decrease ovarian androgen production, improving ovulation
- Enhanced Ovulation: Studies show 50–80% of anovulatory women with PCOS resume ovulation with metformin

- Weight Management Support: Often leads to modest weight loss, which further improves insulin sensitivity
- Inflammation Reduction: Has anti-inflammatory properties that may benefit overall reproductive health
- Improved Pregnancy Outcomes: May reduce miscarriage rates and gestational diabetes risk

Research-Backed Fertility Benefits:
- A landmark study in the *New England Journal of Medicine* found that metformin restored ovulation in 89% of women with PCOS, compared to 12% with placebo[1]
- Multiple studies show metformin can improve IVF outcomes in women with PCOS by enhancing egg quality and reducing ovarian hyperstimulation syndrome risk
- Research demonstrates reduced miscarriage rates when metformin is continued through the first trimester in PCOS patients

Optimal Implementation:
- Starting Dose: Typically 500mg twice daily with meals, gradually increased to 1000mg twice daily
- Extended-Release Formulation: Often better tolerated with fewer GI side effects
- Timing: Best taken with meals to minimize digestive upset
- Duration: Usually continued through conception and often through the first trimester or as long as is needed

---

1   Nestler, J.E., Jakubowicz, D.J., Evans, W.S., Pasquali, R. (1998). Effects of metformin on spontaneous and clomiphene-induced ovulation in the polycystic ovary syndrome. *New England Journal of Medicine*, 338 (26), 1876-1880.

- Monitoring: Regular B12 levels, as metformin can affect B12 absorption (Note: I typically put these patients on a B complex to cover these bases)
- Side Effects: Hypoglycemia or GI distress are the most common

GLP-1 RECEPTOR AGONISTS: THE NEW FRONTIER

GLP-1 (glucagon-like peptide-1) receptor agonists, including medications like semaglutide (Ozempic, Wegovy) and liraglutide (Victoza, Saxenda), represent a newer class of medications that can profoundly impact fertility through multiple mechanisms.

Mechanisms of Action for Fertility:
- Enhanced Insulin Sensitivity: More potent than metformin for improving glucose metabolism
- Significant Weight Loss: Often 10–20% body weight reduction, which dramatically improves fertility in overweight individuals
- Appetite Regulation: Reduces food cravings and portion sizes naturally
- Improved Beta Cell Function: Helps preserve pancreatic insulin-producing cells
- Reduced Inflammation: Systemic anti-inflammatory effects benefit reproductive health
- Cardiovascular Benefits: Improves overall metabolic health, supporting pregnancy

Fertility-Specific Benefits:
- PCOS Management: Particularly effective for women with PCOS and significant weight challenges
- Ovulation Restoration: Weight loss and improved insulin sensitivity often restore regular cycles
- Enhanced IVF Outcomes: Pre-treatment with GLP-1 agonists may improve IVF success rates
- Reduced Pregnancy Complications: Better metabolic health reduces risks of gestational diabetes and hypertension

Important Considerations:
- Discontinuation Timeline: Generally discontinued 2–3 months before conception attempts due to limited pregnancy safety data
- Weight Loss Planning: Rapid weight loss should be completed well before conception attempts
- Nutritional Support: Requires careful attention to nutrition during weight loss phase
- Medical Supervision: Requires ongoing monitoring and dosage adjustments
- Side effects can happen, including: abdominal pain, nausea, hypoglycemia, constipation, and diarrhea

Integration with Functional Medicine Approaches

The most effective approach combines pharmaceutical support with comprehensive lifestyle modifications:

Synergistic Strategies:
1. Enhanced Supplement Absorption: Better insulin sensitivity improves uptake of fertility-supporting nutrients
2. Accelerated Results: Medications can provide faster metabolic improvements while lifestyle changes take effect
3. Sustainable Changes: Pharmaceutical support can make lifestyle modifications easier to maintain
4. Optimized Timing: Use medications to achieve metabolic goals, then transition to maintenance with lifestyle alone

Comprehensive Protocol Example:
- Months 1–3: Begin metformin or GLP-1 agonist alongside anti-inflammatory nutrition and targeted supplementation
- Months 3–6: Achieve metabolic targets (improved insulin sensitivity, weight goals, regular ovulation)
- Month 6+: Transition to conception phase, continuing metformin if appropriate, discontinuing GLP-1 agonists

WHO SHOULD CONSIDER THESE MEDICATIONS?

Metformin Candidates:
- Women with PCOS and insulin resistance
- Individuals with prediabetes or metabolic syndrome
- Those with family history of diabetes
- Women with history of gestational diabetes
- Anyone with elevated fasting insulin levels despite lifestyle modifications

GLP-1 Agonist Candidates:
- Individuals with significant weight to lose (BMI >30)
- Those with insulin resistance not responding adequately to metformin
- People with strong food cravings or appetite dysregulation
- Individuals with cardiovascular risk factors
- Those who have struggled with sustainable weight loss through diet alone

SAFETY CONSIDERATIONS AND MONITORING

Metformin Safety Profile:
- Generally well-tolerated with primarily GI side effects (nausea, diarrhea)
- Rare risk of lactic acidosis in kidney disease
- Can reduce B12 absorption—monitor levels and supplement if needed
- Safe during pregnancy and breastfeeding for appropriate candidates

GLP-1 Agonist Considerations:
- More expensive than metformin
- Injectable medications (though oral forms now available)
- Potential GI side effects, especially initially
- Limited long-term safety data in pregnancy
- Requires careful discontinuation planning before conception

Integration Timeline for Fertility

Pre-Conception Phase (3–6 months before attempting conception):
- Begin appropriate medication under medical supervision
- Implement comprehensive lifestyle modifications simultaneously
- Monitor metabolic markers (glucose, insulin, HbA1c)
- Track fertility markers (cycle regularity, ovulation)

Conception Preparation Phase (1–2 months before attempting conception):
- Discontinue GLP-1 agonists if using
- Continue metformin if appropriate and medically advised
- Optimize all other fertility factors
- Confirm metabolic improvements are maintained

Active Conception Phase:
- Continue metformin if prescribed (often beneficial through first trimester)
- Maintain all lifestyle modifications
- Monitor closely with healthcare team

THE BOTTOM LINE

While supplements and lifestyle modifications should always form the foundation of insulin resistance treatment, pharmaceutical options can provide crucial support for individuals with more significant metabolic challenges. The key is using these medications strategically—as tools to help achieve optimal metabolic health rather than as permanent solutions.

Just as a skilled contractor might use power tools to complete a renovation more efficiently while still requiring proper technique and quality materials, metformin and GLP-1 agonists can accelerate fertility improvements when combined with comprehensive functional medicine approaches.

The goal is always to create sustainable health improvements that support not just conception, but optimal pregnancy outcomes and long-term wellness for both parents and children. These medications, when used appropriately and under proper medical supervision, can be valuable components of a comprehensive fertility optimization strategy.

THE PCOS-FERTILITY CONNECTION

Polycystic ovary syndrome is the most common cause of anovulatory infertility, accounting for up to 80% of cases where women don't ovulate regularly. The good news is that it's also one of the most responsive conditions to proper "electrical system rewiring."
When the hormonal circuitry is rebalanced:
- Follicles can mature properly
- Ovulation can occur predictably
- The uterine lining develops adequately for implantation
- Hormonal support for early pregnancy improves

Unlike endometriosis or some other structural challenges, PCOS doesn't typically damage reproductive organs directly—it primarily disrupts their function through hormonal signaling. This means that when the underlying insulin resistance and inflammation are addressed, fertility often returns without the need for structural interventions.

Of course, age remains an important factor, and women with PCOS shouldn't delay seeking help if pregnancy is desired, as functional rewiring takes time to implement and show results.

AMENORRHEA: INTERRUPTED SUPPLY LINES

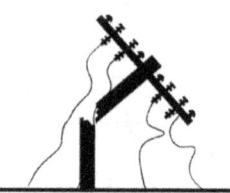

Using our home renovation metaphor, amenorrhea—the absence of menstruation—is like interrupted supply lines to your house. Just as a home needs reliable water, gas, and electrical supplies to function properly, your reproductive system requires consistent hormonal flow and nutrient delivery. When these supply lines become interrupted, your menstrual cycle—the most visible sign of reproductive function—stops flowing altogether.

SYSTEM ANALYSIS: SYMPTOMS AND DIAGNOSIS

Primary Indicators:

Unlike many fertility challenges with numerous symptoms, amenorrhea has one defining characteristic: the absence of menstruation. However, this interruption in service can manifest in different scenarios:

- **Primary Amenorrhea:** When menstruation never begins by age 15 or 16 (the supply lines were never properly connected)
- **Secondary Amenorrhea:** When previously regular periods stop for 3+ consecutive months (the supply lines that once worked have become interrupted)

Associated Warning Signs:

While the absence of periods is the main symptom, you might notice these additional indicators that your body's supply lines are compromised:

- Headaches or vision changes (in some cases)
- Hot flashes or night sweats
- Vaginal dryness
- Excess facial hair growth
- Acne
- Milk discharge from breasts (galactorrhea)
- Changes in voice
- Hair loss or thinning hair

DIAGNOSTIC SYSTEM ANALYSIS:

Diagnosing the cause of amenorrhea is like hiring specialized inspectors to check each potential supply line disruption point:

1. **Comprehensive Health History:**
   - Menstrual history
   - Exercise habits and intensity
   - Dietary patterns and recent weight changes
   - Stress levels and life changes
   - Medications list
   - History of other health conditions

2. **Physical Examination:**
   - Assessment of vital signs
   - Evaluation of height/weight ratio and body composition

- Examination for physical signs of hormone imbalances
- Thyroid examination
- Pelvic examination

3. **Laboratory Tests:**
    - Pregnancy test (the most common cause of interrupted menstruation)
    - Hormone panel: FSH, LH, estradiol, prolactin, thyroid hormones, testosterone
    - Complete blood count to assess overall health
    - Specific tests based on suspected causes

4. **Imaging Studies:**
    - Pelvic ultrasound to examine reproductive structures
    - MRI of the brain if a pituitary issue is suspected
    - Bone density scan if prolonged amenorrhea exists (to check for bone thinning)

COMMON SUPPLY LINE DISRUPTION POINTS:

Amenorrhea stems from interruptions at different points in your hormonal supply chain:

1. **Hypothalamic Amenorrhea:** The command center stops sending signals to produce hormones
    - Often caused by excessive exercise, under-nutrition, stress, or extreme weight loss
    - The brain essentially conserves energy by shutting down reproductive function

2. **Pituitary Issues:** The secondary distribution center malfunctions
    - Prolactinoma (benign tumor that produces excess prolactin)
    - Pituitary damage or disease

3. **Ovarian Factors:** The end-point production facility stops working
    - Premature ovarian insufficiency
    - Polycystic ovary syndrome
    - Ovarian tumors

4. **Structural Issues:** The physical supply lines are damaged or missing
    - Uterine scarring (Asherman's syndrome)
    - Congenital absence of the uterus or vagina
    - Imperforate hymen

5. **Systemic Interruptions:** Whole-body conditions affecting the reproductive system
    - Thyroid dysfunction
    - Adrenal disorders
    - Chronic diseases (celiac disease, inflammatory bowel disease)
    - Certain medications (particularly hormonal contraceptives)

QUICK FIXES VS. SUSTAINABLE INFRASTRUCTURE IMPROVEMENTS

Quick Fixes (Conventional Approach):

The conventional medical approach to amenorrhea often resembles emergency utility repairs that restore service without addressing underlying infrastructure problems:

1. **Hormonal Replacement:**
    - Providing synthetic hormones through birth control pills to induce artificial periods
    - Hormone replacement therapy to mimic natural hormone production
    - These approaches create the appearance of a functioning system without actually restoring natural function

2. **Medication Interventions:**
    - Dopamine agonists for high prolactin levels
    - Clomid or letrozole to induce ovulation when trying to conceive
    - These act like temporary supply boosters rather than permanent repairs

3. **Surgery for Structural Issues:**
    - Removing uterine adhesions
    - Treating anatomical abnormalities
    - While sometimes necessary, these interventions focus only on physical blockages

4. **General Advice Without Support:**
    - "Just gain weight" for those with hypothalamic amenorrhea

- "Reduce stress" without providing tools or resources
- "Exercise less" without addressing the underlying compulsion

While these approaches may restore menstruation or fertility temporarily, they often fail to address why the supply lines were interrupted in the first place.

Sustainable Infrastructure Improvements (Functional Approach): The functional medicine approach seeks to rebuild your body's supply infrastructure from the ground up:

1. **Hypothalamic-Pituitary-Ovarian (HPO) Axis Restoration:**
    - Identifying and removing stressors to the system
    - Supporting communication between the brain and ovaries
    - Key supplements: adaptogenic herbs (ashwagandha, rhodiola), vitamin B complex, magnesium

2. **Metabolic Foundation Rebuilding:**
    - Ensuring adequate caloric intake (often 2000+ calories for active women)
    - Balancing macronutrients with emphasis on healthy fats and high-quality protein
    - Timing nutrition around exercise to minimize energy deficits
    - Critical nutrients: zinc, vitamin A, omega-3 fatty acids

3. **Exercise Recalibration:**
   - Reducing high-intensity training if excessive
   - Incorporating restorative movement like yoga and walking
   - Adding strength training to build metabolic reserve
   - Planning strategic recovery periods

4. **Stress Infrastructure Overhaul:**
   - HPA-axis support through stress reduction techniques
   - Sleep optimization (8+ hours per night)
   - Mindfulness practices and nervous system regulation
   - Setting healthier emotional and psychological boundaries

5. **Nutrient Supply Line Restoration:**
   - Comprehensive micronutrient assessment and repletion
   - Digestive support to ensure proper nutrient absorption
   - Anti-inflammatory nutrition to reduce systemic strain
   - Specific nutrients for hormone production: vitamin D, iodine, selenium

6. **Body Composition Optimization:**
   - Healthy weight restoration for underweight individuals
   - Focus on body composition rather than scale weight
   - Building metabolic reserve through muscle development
   - Addressing disordered eating patterns with professional support

> **Success Story:** Melissa was a 29-year-old marathon runner who hadn't had a period in over two years. Despite multiple doctors telling her this was "normal for athletes," she knew she wanted to start a family soon and was concerned about her fertility. A functional medicine approach revealed significant energy deficits, HPA-axis dysfunction, and low body-fat percentage. By increasing her caloric intake by 600 calories daily, incorporating more rest days, adding specific nutrients (especially zinc, vitamin D, and omega-3s), and working with a therapist on her relationship with exercise, Melissa's period returned within four months. Six months later, she conceived naturally while maintaining a modified running schedule that supported rather than hindered her hormonal health.

However, that sounds easy—too easy—and this is not always the case. I'll expand with some more complex testimonies in the next section on premature ovarian failure.

THE AMENORRHEA-FERTILITY CONNECTION

Amenorrhea is more than an inconvenience—it's a clear signal that your reproductive system lacks the resources to support pregnancy. No menstruation means no ovulation, and without ovulation, conception is impossible.

However, the encouraging news is that amenorrhea is often one of the most reversible causes of infertility when the appropriate approach is taken. When you restore the supply lines:

- The hypothalamus resumes sending GnRH signals
- The pituitary gland responds by releasing FSH and LH
- The ovaries receive these signals and begin follicle development
- Ovulation occurs, followed by the rise in progesterone
- The endometrium builds and sheds appropriately

This restoration process doesn't just enable menstruation—it creates the entire physiological environment needed for conception and healthy pregnancy. Many women find that addressing the root causes of their amenorrhea not only restores their cycles but also improves their overall health, energy, mood, and quality of life.

Unlike conditions that may cause permanent damage to reproductive organs, functional hypothalamic amenorrhea is largely reversible when the body receives the right signals that it's safe to reproduce. The key is patience and consistency—rebuilding supply infrastructure takes time, typically 3–6 months, but can lead to sustainable fertility without ongoing medical intervention.

CHAPTER 12

SYSTEM FAILURES AND TRANSITIONS

PREMATURE OVARIAN FAILURE: EARLY SYSTEM SHUTDOWN

In our home renovation metaphor, premature ovarian failure (POF)—now often referred to as primary ovarian insufficiency (POI)—is like experiencing an early system shutdown in a relatively new home. Imagine if your home's major systems were designed to function reliably for 50+ years, but suddenly began failing after just 20 or 30 years. This is what happens with POF/POI, where the ovaries stop functioning properly before age 40, much earlier than the natural transition to menopause (typically around age 51).

This early shutdown doesn't just affect comfort—it impacts the entire functionality of the home, particularly its ability to support new life.

DIAGNOSTIC INSPECTION: SYMPTOMS AND EARLY WARNING SIGNS

Primary System Failure Indicators:

When your reproductive system experiences premature shutdown, several warning lights may flash:

- **Irregular or Missed Periods:** Often the first sign that ovarian function is declining
- **Hot Flashes and Night Sweats:** Temperature regulation issues similar to menopause
- **Vaginal Dryness:** Decreased estrogen affecting tissue moisture and comfort
- **Sleep Disturbances:** Difficulty falling or staying asleep
- **Irritability or Mood Changes:** Hormonal fluctuations affecting neurotransmitters
- **Decreased Sex Drive:** Libido changes related to hormonal shifts
- **Painful Intercourse:** Due to vaginal dryness and tissue changes
- **Difficulty Concentrating:** Cognitive effects of changing hormone levels
- **Infertility:** Trouble conceiving despite regular attempts

Early Warning Signs Often Missed:

Before complete system shutdown, your body may show subtle signs that are frequently overlooked:

- **Shortened Menstrual Cycles:** Periods coming closer together (every 21–24 days rather than 28)
- **Reduced Menstrual Flow:** Lighter periods than your normal
- **Increased PMS Symptoms:** More intense mood, physical, or cognitive symptoms before periods

- **Unexplained Fatigue:** Beyond normal tiredness, often dismissed as stress
- **Family History Patterns:** Early menopause in female relatives (mother, sisters, aunts)

DIAGNOSTIC INSPECTION PROCESS:
Diagnosing POF/POI involves a comprehensive system inspection:
1. **Medical History Analysis:**
    - Age of first menstruation
    - Pregnancy history
    - Recent changes in menstrual patterns
    - Family history of early menopause
    - Previous ovarian surgery, chemotherapy, or radiation
    - Autoimmune conditions
    - Viral infections
    - Toxin Exposure (even vaccinations)

2. **Physical Examination:**
    - Signs of estrogen deficiency
    - Thyroid assessment
    - Checking for signs of autoimmune conditions

3. **Laboratory Testing:**
    - FSH (follicle-stimulating hormone): Elevated levels (>25 mIU/mL) on two occasions at least one month apart strongly suggest POF
    - Estradiol: Usually low in POF/POI
    - AMH (anti-Müllerian hormone): Measures ovarian reserve
    - Inhibin B: Another marker of ovarian function

- Prolactin: To rule out other causes
- Thyroid function tests: To exclude thyroid disorders
- Autoimmune panels: Checking for associated conditions
- Karyotype: Genetic testing for chromosomal abnormalities
- FMR1 gene testing: For Fragile X premutation

4. **Transvaginal Ultrasound:**
    - Evaluating ovary size (often small in POF)
    - Antral follicle count (typically reduced)
    - Assessing uterine lining thickness

UNDERSTANDING THE CAUSES OF EARLY SHUTDOWN:

POF/POI can result from various factors affecting your reproductive system:

1. **Genetic Factors:** Like faulty wiring installed during construction
    - Chromosomal abnormalities (Turner syndrome, X chromosome deletions)
    - Fragile X premutation
    - Galactosemia
    - Other genetic mutations

2. **Autoimmune Dysfunction:** Your body's defense system attacking its own components
    - Anti-ovarian antibodies
    - Associated with other autoimmune conditions (thyroiditis, Addison's disease, diabetes)

3. **Toxin Exposure:** Environmental damage to the system
   o   Chemotherapy
   o   Radiation therapy
   o   Environmental toxins (especially mold!)
   o   Heavy metals
   o   Cigarette smoke
   o   Vaccinations

4. **Viral Damage:** Infections affecting system integrity
   o   Epstein-Barr
   o   Mumps
   o   Tuberculosis
   o   Shingles virus
   o   Cytomegalovirus

5. **Surgical/Procedural Impact:** Physical damage to the infrastructure
   o   Ovarian surgery
   o   Multiple ovarian biopsies
   o   Endometriosis surgeries
   o   Pelvic damage

6. **Idiopathic:** Unknown causes of system failure (accounts for approximately 50-75% of cases)

EMERGENCY INTERVENTIONS VS. FUNCTIONAL RETROFITTING
Emergency Interventions (Conventional Approach):
The conventional medical approach to POF/POI often resembles emergency system repairs without addressing why the shutdown occurred:

1. **Hormone Replacement Therapy (HRT):**
   - May use birth control pills for younger women or traditional HRT for older women
   - Providing external sources of estrogen and progesterone
   - Typically recommended until the average age of natural menopause, although I recommend this be continued for aging benefits in general
   - Addresses symptoms and protects bone density, cardiovascular health, and cognitive function

2. **Fertility Interventions:**
   - Egg donation with IVF (considered the most effective option)
   - Embryo donation
   - Occasionally, ovulation induction medications (though typically ineffective in true POF)

3. **Symptom Management:**
   - Lubricants and moisturizers for vaginal dryness
   - Sleep aids for insomnia
   - Antidepressants for mood changes
   - Bone-building medications for osteoporosis prevention

4. **Regular Monitoring:**
   - Bone density scans
   - Cardiovascular risk assessments
   - Thyroid function testing
   - Adrenal function evaluation

These approaches primarily focus on replacing what's missing and managing symptoms rather than investigating why the system failed prematurely or whether partial function can be restored.

Functional Retrofitting (Comprehensive Approach):
While conventional medicine often considers POF/POI irreversible, functional medicine explores potential system retrofitting:

1. **Identify and Address Autoimmune Factors:**
    - Comprehensive autoimmune testing beyond standard panels
    - Anti-inflammatory nutrition protocols (elimination of gluten, dairy, and other potential triggers)
    - Gut healing protocols to address intestinal permeability
    - Immune-modulating supplements: vitamin D, omega-3 fatty acids, glutathione precursors
    - Low-dose naltrexone in specific cases

2. **Detoxification System Enhancement:**
    - Identifying toxicities and supporting liver detoxification pathways
    - Reducing ongoing toxin exposure
    - Targeted supplementation: NAC, milk thistle, glutathione, liposomal vitamin C
    - Infrared sauna therapy for toxin elimination
    - Proper hydration and lymphatic support

3. **Mitochondrial Support for Remaining Follicles:**
    - CoQ10 supplementation (usually 600mg daily)
    - PQQ (pyrroloquinoline quinone)

- L-carnitine
- B-complex vitamins, especially B2 and B3
- Alpha-lipoic acid
- Resveratrol

4. **Hormone Balance Optimization:**
   - Bio-identical hormone replacement when appropriate
   - Adrenal support for stress resilience
   - Thyroid optimization (even within "normal" ranges)
   - Chinese herbs with research support: Rehmannia and Epimedium
   - DHEA supplementation with careful monitoring

5. **Nutritional Foundation Rebuilding:**
   - Nutrient-dense whole foods diet
   - Strategic supplementation based on individual testing
   - Key nutrients: zinc, selenium, iodine, magnesium, vitamin E
   - Optimal protein intake for hormonal precursors
   - Phytoestrogen-rich foods when appropriate

6. **Mind-Body Medicine Integration:**
   - Addressing grief and identity issues associated with diagnosis
   - Stress reduction techniques with physiological impact
   - Heart rate variability training
   - Mindfulness practices
   - Community connection and support groups

Success Story: Elena was diagnosed with premature ovarian failure at age 32 after experiencing irregular periods for two years, followed by complete cessation. Her FSH levels were consistently above 40, and her AMH was nearly undetectable. After being told by three reproductive endocrinologists that egg donation was her only option for pregnancy, she worked with a functional medicine practitioner who identified undiagnosed Hashimoto's thyroiditis and a significant heavy metal and mycotoxin burden. After 14 months of intensive autoimmune protocol dietary changes, mycotoxin and metal detoxification, and targeted supplementation including CoQ10 and NAC, infrared sauna therapy, and thyroid optimization, Elena had two menstrual cycles. Though they were irregular, testing during the second cycle confirmed ovulation had occurred. She conceived naturally during her fourth cycle. While not every woman with POF will experience returned fertility, Elena's case demonstrates that sometimes "irreversible" conditions can respond to comprehensive system retrofitting.

THE POF-FERTILITY CONNECTION

POF/POI presents one of the most challenging fertility obstacles, with approximately 5-10% of women experiencing spontaneous pregnancy after diagnosis. Unlike many other reproductive challenges, POF/POI directly impacts the fundamental resource needed for fertility: viable eggs.

The functional approach recognizes several important concepts:

1. **Remaining Potential:** Even after diagnosis, most women with POF/POI still have some follicles remaining—they're just not responding properly to hormonal signals
2. **Fluctuating Function:** POF/POI often includes periods of unpredictable ovarian activity rather than complete shutdown
3. **Individualized Causes:** The underlying reasons for premature shutdown vary greatly between individuals, requiring personalized approaches
4. **Whole-System Impact:** Addressing overall health can sometimes create an environment where remaining follicles function more effectively

For fertility purposes, the window of opportunity for functional interventions is typically greatest within the first 1–2 years after diagnosis, particularly for women whose FSH levels fluctuate rather than remain consistently elevated.

While egg donation remains the most reliable path to pregnancy with POF/POI, the functional approach offers potential alternatives for women who wish to explore them, while simultaneously supporting overall health regardless of fertility outcomes.

PMS/PMDD: CYCLICAL SYSTEM FAILURES

In our home renovation metaphor, premenstrual syndrome (PMS) and its more severe form, called premenstrual dysphoric disorder (PMDD), represent cyclical system failures in your body's infrastructure. Imagine if your home's heating, electrical, and plumbing systems functioned perfectly for three weeks each month, but then predictably malfunctioned during the fourth week—lights flickering, pipes knocking, and temperature fluctuating wildly. This is what happens in PMS/PMDD: recurring physical, emotional, and cognitive symptoms that reliably appear in the luteal phase of your cycle (the days between ovulation and menstruation).

While many women experience mild premenstrual changes, when symptoms significantly disrupt your quality of life or relationships, it signals a deeper hormonal imbalance—one that has critical implications for fertility.

PATTERN RECOGNITION: SYMPTOMS AND DIAGNOSIS

Recognizing the Cyclical Breakdown Pattern:
PMS and PMDD symptoms appear with predictable timing, typically 5–7 days before menstruation and resolving shortly after bleeding begins. This cyclical pattern is the key diagnostic feature.

COMMON SYSTEM FAILURE MANIFESTATIONS:

Physical Symptoms:
- Bloating and water retention
- Breast tenderness and swelling
- Headaches or migraines
- Fatigue and sleep disturbances
- Joint or muscle pain

- Food cravings or appetite changes
- Acne flares

Emotional and Behavioral Symptoms:
- Irritability or anger
- Anxiety or tension
- Mood swings
- Crying spells
- Depression or feelings of hopelessness
- Overwhelm or feeling out of control
- Social withdrawal

Cognitive Symptoms:
- Difficulty concentrating
- Brain fog
- Forgetfulness
- Indecisiveness
- Sleep difficulties

The PMDD Distinction:

While PMS involves mild to moderate symptoms, PMDD represents a more severe system breakdown, characterized by:
- Severe mood disturbances that significantly impair daily functioning
- Marked irritability, anxiety, or depression
- Feeling overwhelmed or out of control
- Symptoms severe enough to impact work, relationships, and quality of life

Diagnostic Pattern Analysis:

Unlike conditions that can be definitively diagnosed with a single test, PMS and PMDD require pattern recognition over time:

1. **Symptom Tracking:**
    - Daily charting of physical, emotional, and cognitive symptoms across 2–3 complete menstrual cycles
    - Rating symptom severity on a scale (1–10)
    - Noting when symptoms begin and end in relation to menstruation

2. **Medical Evaluation:**
    - Comprehensive health history
    - Ruling out other conditions with similar symptoms (thyroid disorders, perimenopause, depression, anxiety disorders)
    - Physical examination

3. **Laboratory Assessment:**
    - Hormone testing (ideally at specific cycle points)
    - Thyroid panel
    - Adrenal function assessment
    - Vitamin D, B12, and other nutrient levels
    - Inflammatory markers

THE PROGESTERONE CONNECTION: THE MISSING LINK

The most significant system malfunction in PMS/PMDD—and its critical connection to fertility—often involves progesterone:

- **Progesterone Insufficiency:** Many women with PMS/PMDD have adequate estrogen but insufficient progesterone during the luteal phase, creating a relative estrogen dominance
- **Luteal Phase Defects:** Short luteal phases (less than 12 days) or inadequate progesterone production after ovulation
- **The Fertility Impact:** This same progesterone deficiency that causes PMS symptoms also:
    - Compromises the endometrial lining's receptivity to implantation
    - Reduces the ability to maintain an early pregnancy
    - Can lead to early miscarriage (often before pregnancy is detected)

In essence, the same hormonal imbalance causing your premenstrual symptoms may directly impact your ability to conceive and maintain pregnancy. Your body's monthly warning signals are meaningful fertility messengers.

TEMPORARY PATCHES VS. PERMANENT INFRASTRUCTURE IMPROVEMENT

Temporary Patches (Conventional Approach):

The conventional medical approach to PMS/PMDD often resembles applying temporary patches to the recurring system failures:

1. **Symptom-Specific Medications:**
    - NSAIDs for pain
    - Diuretics for bloating
    - SSRIs (selective serotonin reuptake inhibitors) for mood symptoms
    - Anti-anxiety medications
    - Sleep aids

2. **Hormonal Interventions:**
   - Birth control pills to suppress ovulation (which also eliminates fertility)
   - Synthetic progestins that don't offer the same benefits as natural progesterone
   - GnRH agonists that create artificial menopause (with significant side effects)

3. **General Lifestyle Advice:**
   - Exercise more
   - Reduce stress
   - Avoid salt, caffeine, and alcohol
   - Get more sleep

While these approaches may provide temporary relief, they frequently mask symptoms without addressing the underlying hormonal imbalances. More concerning for women seeking fertility, many conventional treatments (particularly hormonal birth control) eliminate fertility in the process of managing symptoms.

Permanent Infrastructure Improvement (Functional Approach):
The functional medicine approach seeks to rebuild your hormonal infrastructure for lasting resolution and improved fertility:

1. **Hormone Balancing Strategies:**
   - **Natural Progesterone Support:**
     » Vitex (chasteberry) to enhance pituitary signaling for increased progesterone
     » Vitamin B6 (50–100mg daily) for improved progesterone production

- » Specific seed cycling protocols (pumpkin and flax seeds in follicular phase, sesame and sunflower seeds in luteal phase)
- » Bioidentical oral progesterone when indicated (typically 100–200mg during luteal phase only)

- o **Estrogen Metabolism Support:**
  - » Cruciferous vegetables and DIM (diindolylmethane) supplements
  - » Calcium D-glucarate to support healthy estrogen elimination
  - » Liver support for proper hormone processing
  - » Fiber to ensure removed hormones exit the body

- o **Stress Hormone Regulation:**
  - » Adaptogenic herbs to balance cortisol (ashwagandha, rhodiola, holy basil)
  - » Phosphatidylserine to normalize evening cortisol
  - » Magnesium glycinate or Magnesium L-threonate for nervous system regulation
  - » L-theanine for acute stress response management

2. **Neurotransmitter Support:**
   - o 5-HTP or tryptophan for serotonin support (precursors)
   - o GABA support through specific probiotics and fermented foods
   - o Vitamin B complex for neurotransmitter synthesis

- Inositol (2–4g daily) for improved neurotransmitter receptor sensitivity

3. **Inflammation Reduction:**
   - Anti-inflammatory nutrition (Mediterranean or traditional Asian dietary patterns)
   - Omega-3 supplementation (2–4g daily)
   - Curcumin with enhanced bioavailability
   - Elimination of inflammatory triggers
   - Prioritizing sleep quality for cellular repair

4. **Blood Sugar Stabilization:**
   - Protein-containing meals every 3–4 hours
   - Complex carbohydrates paired with healthy fats
   - Chromium and alpha-lipoic acid for insulin sensitivity
   - Cinnamon and berberine for glucose regulation

5. **Comprehensive Nutrient Repletion:**
   - Magnesium: The master mineral for PMS (400–600mg daily)
   - Vitamin D: Essential for hormone production (typically 2000–5000 IU daily)
   - Calcium: For mood and muscle function (600–1200mg daily)
   - Zinc: Critical for hormone production and immune function (15–30mg daily)
   - B-complex: For hormone metabolism and neurotransmitter support

> **Success Story:** Jasmine suffered from severe PMS for over a decade, with symptoms so debilitating she had to take sick days monthly. Her gynecologist had prescribed birth control pills, which helped somewhat but came with side effects, including decreased libido. When she decided to try conceiving, she stopped taking the pill, and her symptoms returned with greater intensity. Testing revealed significantly low progesterone during her luteal phase and elevated cortisol. After four months of targeted supplementation including Vitex, magnesium, B6, and adaptogens, plus blood sugar stabilizing nutrition, her PMS symptoms reduced by approximately 80%. When she conceived three months later, her functional medicine doctor continued supporting her progesterone levels naturally through the first trimester, and she carried to term without complications.

Note: Not every patient responds successfully to Vitex. I've found that the older my patients are, the greater the likelihood of needing to take bioidentical progesterone.

THE PMS/PMDD-FERTILITY CONNECTION: BUILDING A SUSTAINABLE FOUNDATION

The presence of PMS or PMDD serves as a valuable warning system—your body is signaling hormonal imbalances that may impact fertility in three critical ways:

1. **Compromised Implantation Environment:**
   - Adequate progesterone is essential for proper endometrial development
   - The same progesterone deficiency causing PMS symptoms creates a less receptive uterine lining for implantation
   - Even if fertilization occurs, implantation may fail due to insufficient luteal support

2. **Early Pregnancy Vulnerability:**
   - Progesterone maintains pregnancy until the placenta takes over at around 10–12 weeks
   - Low progesterone may lead to early miscarriage, often before pregnancy is detected
   - These can appear as slightly late, heavy periods rather than recognized pregnancies

3. **Hormonal Foundation for Pregnancy:**
   - Progesterone levels during pregnancy should rise steadily
   - Women with pre-existing progesterone insufficiency often struggle to maintain adequate levels
   - This can lead to complications including recurrent miscarriage and preterm labor

The good news is that addressing the root causes of PMS/PMDD not only relieves monthly symptoms but simultaneously creates the optimal hormonal environment for conception and pregnancy. By fixing the cyclical system failures rather than masking them, you build a stronger infrastructure for bringing new life into your home.

When working with women experiencing both PMS/PMDD and fertility challenges, I've observed that resolving the hormonal imbalances causing premenstrual symptoms frequently leads to improved fertility outcomes. The timeline typically involves:

- 1–2 cycles: Initial symptom improvement
- 3–4 cycles: Significant PMS/PMDD symptom reduction
- 4–6 cycles: Optimized hormonal patterns supporting fertility

Rather than viewing PMS/PMDD as a separate issue from fertility, recognize it as a connected part of your reproductive health system—when you resolve the monthly breakdowns, you're simultaneously building a stronger foundation for conception and pregnancy.

PERIMENOPAUSE/MENOPAUSE: SYSTEM TRANSITIONS

In our home renovation metaphor, perimenopause and menopause represent a major system transition—similar to converting an outdated electrical system to a new configuration. This isn't a malfunction but rather a natural evolution of your reproductive infrastructure. However, just as with any significant home upgrade, this transition can either be smooth and well-managed or disruptive and chaotic.

For women approaching or experiencing these changes while still hoping to conceive, understanding this transition is crucial—because while the window is narrowing, opportunities may still exist with the right approach.

RECOGNIZING THE REMODELING PHASE: SYMPTOMS AND DIAGNOSIS

Understanding the Transition Timeline:
- **Perimenopause:** The transitional years leading up to menopause (typically starting in early to mid-40s, but sometimes as early as late 30s)
- **Menopause:** Officially diagnosed after 12 consecutive months without a menstrual period (average age 51 in the U.S.)
- **Postmenopause:** The years following menopause

System Transition Indicators:

During perimenopause, your body begins switching from a cyclical reproductive system to a new configuration. This remodeling process often creates noticeable changes:

Menstrual Changes:
- Irregular cycles (shorter, longer, or unpredictable)
- Changes in flow (heavier, lighter, or fluctuating)
- Skipped periods
- Shorter cycles (may shorten to 21–25 days)

Hormonal Fluctuation Signs:
- Hot flashes and night sweats
- Sleep disturbances
- Mood changes (irritability, anxiety, depression)
- Vaginal dryness
- Decreased libido
- Increased PMS symptoms
- Brain fog or memory issues
- Weight redistribution (especially around the abdomen)

- Skin changes (dryness, thinning)
- Hair changes (thinning, texture changes)

Fertility Indication Signs:
- Greater difficulty conceiving
- Cycles where ovulation doesn't occur
- Shortened luteal phase
- More pronounced follicular phase symptoms

DIAGNOSTIC ASSESSMENT:

Identifying where you are in the perimenopause-to-menopause transition involves:

1. **Symptom Evaluation:**
    - Tracking menstrual cycle changes
    - Documenting vasomotor symptoms (hot flashes, night sweats)
    - Noting sleep patterns and quality
    - Monitoring mood and cognitive changes

2. **Hormone Testing:**
    - FSH (follicle-stimulating hormone): Levels begin rising as ovaries become less responsive
    - Estradiol: Often fluctuates dramatically during perimenopause before declining
    - Progesterone: often the first hormone to decline and the first to need replaced
    - AMH (anti-Müllerian hormone): Provides insight into remaining ovarian reserve
    - Inhibin B: Another marker of ovarian function in women (and Sertoli cell function in men) that declines with age

- Thyroid function: Often changes during this transition

3. **Ovarian Reserve Assessment:**
    - Transvaginal ultrasound for antral follicle count
    - Comprehensive hormone panels at specific cycle days
    - Tracking ovulation through basal body temperature or ovulation predictor kits

The challenge in diagnosing perimenopause is that it's a dynamic process, not a single point in time. Hormone levels often fluctuate dramatically—you might have an FSH reading of 25 one month (suggesting declining ovarian function) and 10 the next month (appearing more premenopausal). This variability reflects the underlying system transition.

STANDARD UPGRADES VS. CUSTOMIZED RENOVATION APPROACHES

Standard Upgrades (Conventional Approach):
The conventional medical approach to perimenopause often involves standardized interventions without much customization:

1. **Hormone Replacement Therapy (HRT):**
    - One-size-fits-all dosing of synthetic hormones
    - Primarily focused on symptom relief rather than optimizing remaining fertility
    - Often discouraged until after complete menopause

2. **Symptom-Specific Medications:**
    - Antidepressants for mood changes
    - Sleep medications for insomnia
    - Osteoporosis medications for bone density concerns
    - Vaginal estrogen for local symptoms

3. **Fertility Assessment:**
   - Often pessimistic outlook for natural conception
   - Quick recommendation for donor eggs or adoption
   - Limited exploration of remaining fertility potential

4. **General Lifestyle Advice:**
   - Exercise more
   - Reduce stress
   - Maintain a healthy weight
   - Limited nutritional guidance

For women specifically interested in fertility during this transition, conventional approaches typically offer limited options—either pursuing aggressive fertility treatments immediately or accepting diminished chances of conception.

CUSTOMIZED RENOVATION APPROACHES (FUNCTIONAL PERSPECTIVE):

The functional medicine approach recognizes that this system transition can be optimized through personalized interventions:

1. **Hormonal Orchestration:**
   - **Bioidentical Hormone Support:** Individualized hormone prescriptions based on specific deficiencies
   - **Progesterone Emphasis:** Often the first hormone to decline, supporting with bioidentical progesterone can improve cycle quality and fertility
   - **Testosterone Consideration:** Low levels impact energy, libido, and egg quality
   - **Pregnenolone and DHEA:** Precursor hormones that support overall hormone production

- Cycle-Matching Protocols: Varying supplements and support throughout the menstrual cycle

2. **Ovarian Reserve Optimization:**
   - **Mitochondrial Support:** CoQ10 (typically 600mg daily), PQQ, NAC, resveratrol
   - **Antioxidant Protection:** Melatonin, vitamin E (as mixed tocopherols), vitamin C, glutathione
   - **Anti-glycation Strategies:** Alpha-lipoic acid, berberine, cinnamon
     » These aim to combat glycation, a natural process where sugars bind to proteins, potentially leading to damage and aging.
   - **Targeted Nutrition:** Higher protein intake, strategic carbohydrate timing, increased healthy fats

3. **Inflammation Management:**
   - **Anti-inflammatory Diet:** Mediterranean, traditional Asian, or custom elimination protocol
   - **Key Supplements:** Specialized turmeric formulations, omega-3 fatty acids, SPMs (specialized pro-resolving mediators)
   - **Stress Reduction Protocols:** Tailored to individual patterns and preferences
   - **Sleep Optimization:** Supporting the body's primary recovery mechanism

4. **Metabolic Efficiency:**
   - **Insulin Sensitivity Enhancement:** Berberine, magnesium, chromium, zinc

- **Exercise Prescription:** Strength training, zone 2 cardiovascular training, and recovery strategies
- **Glucose Regulation:** Continuous glucose monitoring for personalized nutrition
- **Strategic Fasting Protocols:** Tailored to hormonal status and goals

5. **Detoxification Support:**
   - **Estrogen Metabolism:** DIM, calcium D-glucarate, broccoli seed extract
   - **Liver Function Optimization:** Milk thistle, artichoke extract, amino acid precursors
   - **Environmental Toxin Reduction:** Home environment assessment and remediation
   - **Personalized Detox Pathways:** Based on genetic testing and functional assessment

> **Success Story:** Margot sought out functional medicine at age 44 after being told by three reproductive endocrinologists that her only path to pregnancy was donor eggs. Her FSH fluctuated between 15-23, and her AMH was 0.3 ng/mL—indicators of diminished ovarian reserve. Rather than immediately pursuing donor eggs, she implemented a comprehensive four-month preparation protocol after testing her for nutritional deficiencies of CoQ10

> (600mg daily), melatonin (3mg at bedtime), DHEA (under careful monitoring), strategic protein timing, and bioidentical progesterone support in her luteal phase. While still considered high-risk due to her age, Margot conceived naturally in her fifth cycle. She maintained the pregnancy with continued progesterone support and delivered a healthy baby girl just before her 45th birthday.

THE PERIMENOPAUSE-FERTILITY CONNECTION: MAKING THE MOST OF TRANSITION TIME

The perimenopausal transition presents both challenges and opportunities for fertility:

Fertility Challenges During System Transition:
1. **Egg Quality Concerns:**
    - Mitochondrial dysfunction increases with age
    - DNA repair mechanisms become less efficient
    - Oxidative damage accumulates
    - Chromosomal abnormalities become more common

2. **Ovulatory Irregularities:**
    - Some cycles may be anovulatory (no egg released)
    - Ovulation timing becomes less predictable
    - Follicular development may be suboptimal
    - Luteal phase often shortens

3. **Hormonal Support Issues:**
    - Progesterone production typically declines first
    - Estrogen fluctuates wildly before declining
    - Testosterone levels affect egg development
    - HPA axis (stress response system) often becomes dysregulated

4. **Uterine Receptivity Changes:**
    - Endometrial lining may become thinner
    - Blood flow to the uterus may decrease
    - Implantation factors can be altered
    - Increased risk of early pregnancy loss

THE WINDOW OF OPPORTUNITY:

Despite these challenges, the perimenopausal transition offers a critical window of opportunity:

1. **Remaining Follicles:** Even with diminished ovarian reserve, most perimenopausal women still have some viable follicles
2. **Quality Optimization:** While quantity decreases, the quality of remaining eggs can often be improved through targeted interventions
3. **Hormonal Variability:** The fluctuating nature of perimenopause means some cycles are more fertile than others
4. **Responsive Systems:** The body's systems are still adaptable and can respond to appropriate interventions

For women in perimenopause who desire pregnancy, the functional approach focuses on:

- Identifying and maximizing the most fertile cycles
- Improving the quality of remaining eggs rather than lamenting their diminished quantity
- Optimizing the hormonal environment for both conception and pregnancy maintenance
- Addressing the unique challenges of "advanced maternal age" with targeted protocols

BEYOND NATURAL CONCEPTION: INTEGRATIVE APPROACHES

For women whose perimenopausal status makes natural conception unlikely despite optimizations:

1. **Fertility Treatment Preparation:** Using functional approaches to improve outcomes of IVF or other assisted reproductive technologies
2. **Hormone Optimization Before Procedures:** Creating the ideal hormonal environment before undergoing fertility procedures
3. **Support Through Donor Processes:** Preparing the body optimally for donor egg implementation
4. **Whole-Person Preparation for Parenthood:** Focusing on overall health optimization for the demands of pregnancy and parenting at an older age

The perimenopausal transition doesn't mean the end of fertility for all women—but it does require a sophisticated, individualized approach that honors both the challenges and possibilities of this natural system upgrade.

CHAPTER 13

HIDDEN STRUCTURAL PROBLEMS AND CIRCULATION ISSUES

MALE FERTILITY ISSUES: SUPPORT STRUCTURE WEAKNESSES
THE OVERLOOKED HALF OF THE EQUATION

Despite men contributing to approximately 50% of fertility problems, statistics reveal a troubling gap in male evaluation during conception attempts. Only about 20% of men undergo any fertility workup when couples are struggling to conceive, leaving a significant portion of potential issues undiagnosed and untreated.

A comprehensive male fertility evaluation should include several key components. A thorough medical and reproductive history can reveal past infections, injuries, medications, or lifestyle factors that may impact fertility. The physical examination allows assessment of anatomical abnormalities, varicoceles, or signs of hormonal imbalances that could affect sperm production.

Laboratory testing forms the cornerstone of male fertility assessment. A detailed sperm analysis evaluates count, motility, and morphology, while DNA fragmentation testing reveals the genetic integrity of sperm—crucial information that standard sperm analysis cannot provide. Blood work can identify hormonal imbalances, genetic conditions, or underlying health issues affecting reproductive function.

Male anatomy presents unique considerations that make comprehensive evaluation essential. Since everything "comes out the same hole"—the urethra serves as the pathway for both urine and semen—urinary tract infections, prostate infections, and sexually transmitted diseases can all directly impact fertility. These conditions can alter sperm quality, block reproductive pathways, or create inflammatory environments hostile to sperm survival. This anatomical reality underscores why screening for UTIs, prostate issues, and STDs must be integral components of any thorough male fertility workup.

LET'S TALK ABOUT POWERFUL SWIMMERS

From the millions of sperm that begin the journey, these microscopic swimmers possess an extraordinary sense of smell—like sharks detecting blood in the water—that guides them toward their target. They must first survive the hostile environment of the vagina and evade the woman's immune system, which treats them as foreign invaders. The sperm face a narrow window of opportunity: the cervix, which normally maintains a protective barrier to prevent infection from reaching the peritoneum, opens only a few days each month as cervical mucus thins during ovulation. Those that make it through must then swim the equivalent of a human running twenty miles, completing this herculean journey in just minutes.

When the single successful sperm finally penetrates the egg's protective barriers, the egg releases a dramatic burst of zinc ions known as the "zinc spark"—a brilliant flash that marks the spark of life itself. Simultaneously, the egg's membrane undergoes rapid depolarization as calcium voltage channels activate, creating an electrical and chemical barrier that immediately blocks any additional sperm from entering. This remarkable defense mechanism ensures that only one sperm contributes its genetic material, preserving the precise chromosome number needed for healthy development and marking the beginning of a new organism.

MALE FERTILITY ISSUES: SUPPORT STRUCTURE WEAKNESSES

In our home renovation metaphor, male fertility represents the essential support structure of your fertility blueprint. Just as a house needs a solid foundation, reliable framing, and proper structural support to withstand challenges and sustain life within, successful conception requires healthy sperm that can effectively reach and fertilize an egg.

When male fertility issues arise, it's similar to discovering weaknesses in your home's foundational elements—problems that may not be immediately visible but can significantly impact the entire structure's integrity and function.

FOUNDATION INSPECTION: SPERM COUNT AND MOTILITY

Key Structural Elements to Assess:

A comprehensive male fertility evaluation examines several crucial components:

Sperm Production (Count):
- **Normal Range:** 15–200 million sperm per milliliter
- **Oligospermia:** Low sperm count (below 15 million/mL)
- **Azoospermia:** No sperm present in the ejaculate

Sperm Movement (Motility):
- **Progressive Motility:** Percentage of sperm moving efficiently forward (normal: at least 32%)
- **Non-progressive Motility:** Movement without forward progression
- **Immotility:** No movement

Sperm Structure (Morphology):
- **Normal Forms:** Percentage of sperm with proper shape and structure (normal: at least 4%)
- **Head Defects:** Issues with the sperm head containing DNA
- **Midpiece Abnormalities:** Problems with the energy-producing section
- **Tail Defects:** Issues affecting movement capability

Semen Quality Factors:
- **Volume:** Amount of ejaculate (normal: 1.5–5 mL)
- **Liquefaction:** Ability to change from gel to liquid state
- **pH:** Acidity/alkalinity balance (normal: 7.2–8.0)
- **White Blood Cells:** Indicators of infection or inflammation

DNA Integrity:
- **Fragmentation Rate:** Percentage of sperm with DNA damage (ideally below 25%)
- **Chromatin Maturity:** Proper packaging of genetic material

THE INSPECTION PROCESS:

A thorough male fertility assessment typically involves:

1. **Complete Medical History:**
    - Past illnesses and surgeries
    - Medication usage
    - Environmental and occupational exposures
    - Lifestyle factors (smoking nicotine and marijuana, alcohol, exercise, heat exposure)
    - Family history of fertility issues

2. **Physical Examination:**
    - Testicular size and consistency
    - Presence of varicoceles (enlarged veins)
    - Evaluation of the vas deferens and epididymis
    - Secondary sexual characteristics

3. **Semen Analysis:**
    - Basic parameters (count, motility, morphology)
    - Usually repeated 2–3 months apart due to sperm cycle length
    - Best performed after 2–5 days of abstinence

4. **Advanced Testing (When Indicated):**
    - Sperm DNA fragmentation testing
    - Genetic testing for chromosomal abnormalities
    - Hormone panel (testosterone, FSH, LH, estradiol, prolactin)
    - Ultrasound of testes and prostate
    - Specialized functional tests

UNDERSTANDING THE FOUNDATION WEAKNESSES:

Male fertility challenges can stem from various structural issues:

1. **Production Problems:**
    - Hormonal imbalances affecting sperm production
    - Testicular damage or developmental issues
    - Varicoceles affecting temperature regulation
    - Genetic factors influencing sperm development

2. **Transport Blockages:**
    - Obstructions in the epididymis or vas deferens
    - Previous infections causing scarring
    - Congenital absence of the vas deferens
    - Ejaculatory duct obstructions

3. **Delivery Difficulties:**
    - Erectile dysfunction
    - Ejaculation problems (retrograde ejaculation, anejaculation)
    - Anatomical issues such as hypospadias

4. **Quality Control Issues:**
    - DNA fragmentation from oxidative stress
    - Chromosomal abnormalities
    - Immature sperm cells
    - Antibody formation against sperm

STRUCTURAL DAMAGE FROM PAST EVENTS: WHEN PROTECTIVE BARRIERS FAIL

Just as a home's foundation can be compromised by past flooding, earthquakes, or other catastrophic events that weren't apparent during the initial construction, male fertility can be permanently affected by viral infections that occurred years or even decades earlier.

The testicles are protected by a specialized blood-testis barrier, similar to the blood-brain barrier that shields the brain. This selective barrier prevents most substances and pathogens from reaching the delicate sperm-producing cells within the seminiferous tubules. However, certain viruses can breach this protective shield with potentially devastating consequences for male fertility.

The mumps virus presents one of the most significant threats to male reproductive health. This virus, which typically causes swelling of the parotid glands (salivary glands near the ears), can migrate to the testicles, particularly when infection occurs during or after puberty. Mumps orchitis, as this testicular inflammation is known, can cause severe swelling, pain, and potential permanent damage to the sperm-producing tissue. In some cases, this can lead to reduced sperm production or complete sterility in the affected testicle.

The timing of mumps infection is critical—while pre-pubertal boys may experience testicular involvement, the risk of permanent fertility damage is much lower because sperm production hasn't yet begun. However, post-pubertal males face a significant risk of lasting reproductive consequences, so some believe the mumps vaccination is an essential component of protecting future fertility. However, this vaccination does not come without risk. Some believe the vaccination risks are higher than those of the mumps (topic for another book).

CRITICAL MALE FERTILITY PRECAUTIONS: THE HIDDEN SPERM KILLERS

Just as a home renovation requires avoiding certain materials and practices that could compromise the structure, optimizing male fertility demands awareness of specific factors that can dramatically impact sperm production and quality. These often-overlooked considerations can make the difference between successful conception and continued struggles.

THE FATHER'S ENVIRONMENTAL LEGACY

Believe it or not, the father is more likely to pass on environmental stressors through the sperm than previously understood. Research reveals that different types of environmental exposures create distinct patterns of damage:

- **Low motility** typically suggests exposure to short-term toxins like hot baths, saunas, or acute chemical exposure
- **Low count** often indicates chronic toxic exposures from ongoing environmental factors like chemicals, radiation, or dietary contaminants

This environmental impact extends far beyond conception. Babies are most susceptible to these inherited environmental stressors during the first few months of life, when their developing systems are most vulnerable. One particularly concerning study found that women who consumed high amounts of non-organic commercial beef (high in synthetic estrogens) and breastfed their infants had children who later developed low sperm counts in adulthood—demonstrating how environmental toxins can affect fertility across generations.

This multigenerational impact underscores why male fertility optimization isn't just about achieving pregnancy, but about ensuring the long-term reproductive health of future children.

Chemical-Treated Underwear: The Invisible Threat

Many men unknowingly expose their reproductive organs to sperm-damaging chemicals through everyday clothing choices. Conventional underwear often contains:

- Flame retardants that disrupt hormone function
- Antibacterial treatments containing triclosan and other endocrine disruptors
- Fabric treatments with formaldehyde and other reproductive toxins
- Synthetic dyes that can contain heavy metals

These chemicals sit directly against the scrotum for 12+ hours daily, creating constant low-level exposure that can:

- Reduce sperm count and motility
- Increase DNA fragmentation
- Disrupt testosterone production
- Contribute to oxidative stress in reproductive tissues

Solution: Switch to organic cotton or bamboo underwear without chemical treatments. Look for brands that specifically advertise "chemical-free" or "organic" options. This simple change can significantly reduce daily toxin exposure to reproductive organs.

Heat Exposure: Temperature Matters More Than You Think

The testicles hang outside the body for a crucial reason—optimal sperm production requires temperatures 2–4 degrees below core body temperature. Even temporary overheating can damage sperm that won't be released for 74 days.

Critical Heat Sources to Avoid:
- Saunas and hot tubs: Completely avoid during the 3–4 months before attempting conception
- Hot baths: Keep water temperature under 98°F and limit to 15 minutes
- Heated car seats: Use sparingly, especially during long drives
- Laptop computers: Never place directly on lap; use a cooling pad and table (and ideally an EMF blocking pad)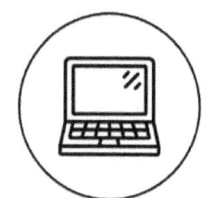
- Tight-fitting pants: Can trap heat and reduce air circulation
- Extended sitting: Take breaks every 30–60 minutes to allow cooling

Many men don't realize that the infrared saunas they use for general health benefits can be counterproductive during fertility optimization. While beneficial for detoxification at other times, the heat exposure during the conception period can significantly impact sperm quality.

ELECTROMAGNETIC FIELD (EMF) EXPOSURE: THE MODERN FERTILITY THREAT

Our modern world exposes us to unprecedented levels of electromagnetic radiation that can directly damage sperm at the cellular level. Research consistently shows that EMF exposure can:
- Reduce sperm motility by up to 25% with regular cell phone use
- Increase DNA fragmentation in sperm, leading to higher miscarriage rates

- Decrease sperm concentration and overall count
- Disrupt mitochondrial function in sperm cells, reducing their energy and viability
- Generate reactive oxygen species that damage sperm membranes and DNA

Major EMF Sources Affecting Male Fertility:
- Cell phones: Never carry in front pockets near reproductive organs
- Laptops and tablets: Always use on a table with proper ventilation; never directly on lap
- Wi-Fi routers: Keep out of bedrooms; consider turning off at night
- Bluetooth devices: Limit use of wireless earbuds and speakers near the body
- Smart watches and fitness trackers: Consider removing during sleep (although I strongly feel 100% avoidance is best)
- Electric blankets: Avoid use, especially during winter months
- Microwave ovens: Maintain distance while operating; check door seals regularly

EMF Protection Strategies:
- Keep cell phones in airplane mode or away from the body when not in use
- Use wired headphones instead of Bluetooth for calls
- Place laptops on desks or use EMF-blocking pads
- Turn off Wi-Fi routers at night or use timer switches

- Create an EMF-free bedroom environment for optimal sleep and hormone production
- Consider EMF meter testing in your home to identify high-exposure areas
- Use speaker phone or wired headsets for longer calls

TESTOSTERONE REPLACEMENT THERAPY: THE FERTILITY PARADOX

This is perhaps the most critical and counterintuitive factor affecting male fertility today. Many men begin testosterone replacement therapy (TRT) to address symptoms like low energy, reduced libido, or mood changes—not realizing it can completely shut down natural sperm production.

How TRT Affects Fertility:
- External testosterone signals the body to stop producing its own testosterone
- This suppresses FSH and LH production from the pituitary gland
- Without FSH and LH signals, the testicles stop producing sperm
- Sperm count can drop to zero within 3–6 months of starting TRT
- This effect can persist for months or even years after discontinuing TRT

The Six-Month Rule: If you're currently on testosterone replacement therapy and planning to conceive, you must:
- Discontinue TRT at least six months before attempting conception, or bank sperm ahead of time

- Work with a knowledgeable physician to support natural testosterone recovery
- Consider alternative approaches to address the symptoms that led to TRT
- Monitor hormone levels throughout the recovery process

Recovery Support Strategies:
- hCG therapy to stimulate natural testosterone production
- Clomiphene citrate to restore pituitary signaling
- Comprehensive nutritional support for hormone production
- Lifestyle modifications to naturally boost testosterone
- Regular monitoring of sperm parameters during recovery

There are ways to preserve testicle size and fertility while on testosterone using the above-mentioned Clomid, but this needs to be done under close supervision of a specialist. We'll be addressing more of this in my next book (spoiler alert).

Important note: Never discontinue TRT without medical supervision. Work with a healthcare provider experienced in fertility and hormone optimization to create a safe transition plan.

SPERM BANKING CONSIDERATIONS

While testosterone replacement therapy remains an important treatment option, men should also consider sperm banking in certain circumstances. Banking sperm is a straightforward, well-established procedure that's been available for decades—far simpler and more affordable than the newer technology of egg freezing for women.

Beyond fertility preservation during TRT, men may want to bank sperm for several other important reasons:

- **Before cancer treatment:** Chemotherapy and radiation can significantly impact sperm production and quality, making sperm banking essential before beginning treatment.

- **Proactive fertility planning:** Younger men without current partners may choose to preserve their highest-quality sperm, similar to how women increasingly freeze eggs in their twenties and thirties. Since sperm quality naturally declines with age, banking sperm at a younger age ensures access to healthier genetic material for future family planning.

- **High-risk occupations:** Men with careers involving exposure to chemicals, radiation, or other reproductive toxins may benefit from banking sperm before prolonged exposures.

PRACTICAL IMPLEMENTATION TIMELINE

For men preparing for conception, implement these changes according to the sperm development cycle:

Months 1–3 Before Conception Attempts:
- Switch to organic, chemical-free underwear
- Discontinue testosterone replacement therapy (with medical supervision)
- Eliminate sauna and hot tub use
- Implement heat-reduction strategies (loose clothing, cooling breaks)
- Minimize EMF exposure (phone away from body, laptop on table, Wi-Fi off at night)

Month 2–3:
- Monitor improvements in energy, libido, and overall well-being as natural hormone production recovers
- Consider sperm analysis to track improvements
- Continue all heat-reduction and chemical-avoidance strategies

Month 3+:
- Optimal window for conception attempts
- Continue all protective strategies (heat reduction, chemical avoidance, EMF minimization)
- Consider follow-up sperm analysis to confirm improvements

Remember that sperm take approximately 74 days to develop fully, so the changes you make today will be reflected in sperm quality 2–3 months from now. This timeline makes consistency crucial—even occasional heat exposure or chemical contact during this period can impact the sperm being developed for future release.

These may seem like small details in your overall fertility journey, but they represent low-hanging fruit that can make a significant difference in outcomes. Just as attention to detail distinguishes a professional renovation from amateur work, addressing these often-overlooked factors can be the difference between continued fertility struggles and successful conception.

QUICK REINFORCEMENT VS. COMPLETE STRUCTURAL ENHANCEMENT
Quick Reinforcement (Conventional Approach):
The conventional medical approach to male fertility often focuses on rapid interventions without addressing underlying structural weaknesses:

1. **Medication Interventions:**
   - Clomiphene citrate to boost testosterone and sperm production
   - hCG (human chorionic gonadotropin) injections
   - Antibiotics for suspected infections
   - Medications for erectile dysfunction

2. **Surgical Procedures:**
   - Varicocele repair (though benefits can take 3–6 months to manifest)
   - Surgical sperm retrieval methods:
     » TESE (testicular sperm extraction)
     » MESA (microsurgical epididymal sperm aspiration)
     » PESA (percutaneous epididymal sperm aspiration)

3. **Assisted Reproductive Technologies:**
   - Intrauterine insemination (IUI) for mild male factor infertility
   - In vitro fertilization (IVF) for moderate issues
   - Intracytoplasmic sperm injection (ICSI) for severe male factor infertility
   - Use of donor sperm when no viable sperm can be obtained

4. **General Lifestyle Advice:**
   - Quit smoking
   - Reduce alcohol
   - Lose weight
   - Avoid hot tubs

While these approaches may provide workable solutions for conception, they often bypass the opportunity to improve overall male health and address the root causes of fertility challenges.

COMPLETE STRUCTURAL ENHANCEMENT (FUNCTIONAL APPROACH):

The functional medicine approach focuses on comprehensive rebuilding of male reproductive health:

1. **Hormonal Foundation Optimization:**
    - **Testosterone Support:** Weight training, vitamin D optimization, zinc, magnesium
    - **Estrogen Balance:** Reducing environmental xenoestrogens, supporting healthy metabolism
    - **Thyroid Optimization:** Comprehensive thyroid testing and support
    - **Stress Hormone Management:** Cortisol rhythm normalization, adaptogenic herbs
    - **Aromatase Activity:** Adjusting when needed with natural compounds like chrysin and zinc

2. **Anti-Inflammatory Construction:**
    - **Inflammatory Foods Removal:** Personalized elimination of reactive foods
    - **Omega Balance Restoration:** Increasing omega-3s, reducing omega-6s
    - **Gut Health Rebuilding:** Probiotics, prebiotic fiber, intestinal permeability support
    - **Key Supplements:** Specialized curcumin formulations, omega-3 fatty acids, boswellia

3. **Oxidative Stress Protection:**
   - **Antioxidant Protocol:** CoQ10 (200–600mg daily), vitamin E (as mixed tocopherols), vitamin C
   - **Glutathione Support:** NAC, milk thistle, alpha-lipoic acid
   - **Mitochondrial Enhancement:** PQQ, D-ribose, L-carnitine
   - **Environmental Toxin Reduction:** Heavy metals assessment, plastics avoidance

4. **Nutritional Density Enhancement:**
   - **Micronutrient Optimization:** Based on individual testing
   - **Key Sperm-Supporting Nutrients:**
     » Zinc (25–50mg daily): Essential for testosterone and sperm production
     » Selenium (100–200mcg daily): Critical for sperm development
     » Folate (400–800mcg daily): Supports DNA integrity
     » L-arginine (2–4g daily): Improves sperm count and motility
     » L-carnitine (2–3g daily): Enhances sperm energy and motility
     » Lycopene (10–30mg daily): Protects developing sperm

5. **Toxin Removal System:**
    - **Endocrine Disruptor Avoidance:** Removing plastics, pesticides, and chemical exposures
    - **Heavy Metal Detection and Removal:** Testing and evidence-based detoxification when indicated
    - **Liver Function Enhancement:** Targeted botanical support
    - **Electromagnetic Field (EMF) Reduction:** Minimizing laptop heat and cell phone proximity

> **Success Story:** Michael and his wife had been trying to conceive for two years without success. Semen analysis showed low count (8 million/mL), poor motility (18% progressive), and elevated DNA fragmentation (38%). Conventional treatment recommended immediate IVF with ICSI. Instead, Michael chose to pursue a three-month functional protocol first: comprehensive nutrient repletion (focusing on zinc, selenium, CoQ10), removal of all alcohol and processed foods, daily moderate exercise, twice-weekly infrared sauna sessions, and stress management through meditation. His follow-up semen analysis showed dramatic improvements: count increased to 28 million/mL, progressive motility rose to 42%, and DNA fragmentation dropped to 22%. The couple conceived naturally within the next 3 months.

THE MALE FACTOR-FERTILITY CONNECTION: EQUAL PARTNERSHIP IN THE BLUEPRINT

Male fertility represents approximately 50% of the conception equation, contributing essential elements to:

1. **Fertilization Success:**
   - Sperm must navigate the female reproductive tract
   - They must have sufficient energy for the journey
   - They need properly functioning enzymes to penetrate the egg
   - DNA must be intact for proper embryo development

2. **Embryo Development:**
   - Paternal DNA influences early cellular division
   - Sperm contribute mitochondrial factors affecting energy production
   - Epigenetic factors from the father impact gene expression
   - Specific genes from the father drive placental development

3. **Pregnancy Health:**
   - Paternal factors influence placentation and implantation
   - Sperm quality affects miscarriage risk
   - Genetic integrity impacts congenital issues
   - Paternal age and health affect pregnancy outcomes

THE FUNCTIONAL ADVANTAGE FOR MALE FERTILITY:

The male reproductive system offers several advantages for fertility enhancement:

1. **Continuous Production:** Unlike women's fixed egg supply, men continuously produce new sperm
2. **Rapid Renewal:** The complete sperm development cycle takes approximately 74 days, meaning positive changes can manifest relatively quickly
3. **Responsive to Intervention:** Sperm quality often shows significant improvement with targeted lifestyle and nutritional interventions
4. **Measurable Outcomes:** Regular semen analysis provides concrete feedback on intervention effectiveness

THE PARTNER PARTICIPATION FACTOR

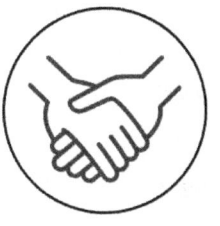

In my clinical practice, I've observed a pattern worth noting: I don't often see male patients who specifically come to me with known fertility issues. However, I've found that couples where the male partner actively participates in the process—attending appointments with their female partner and embracing nutritional and lifestyle optimizations alongside her—typically conceive faster than couples where the male partner is resistant to acknowledging his role in the fertility journey.

This observation highlights an important truth: fertility is truly a *shared* project, much like renovating a home together. When both partners recognize their contribution to the blueprint and actively participate in the renovation process, the project typically progresses more smoothly and successfully.

Even when male fertility parameters appear normal on standard testing, the subtle improvements that come from nutritional optimization, toxin reduction, stress management, and other functional approaches can make a significant difference in conception rates and pregnancy outcomes. A willing male partner who embraces these changes not only improves the chances of conception but also demonstrates the emotional support and partnership that will be essential throughout pregnancy and parenthood.

For couples facing fertility challenges, addressing the male component through comprehensive functional approaches offers a significant opportunity—often with benefits extending beyond fertility to overall health and longevity. Rather than viewing male factor infertility as simply a technical obstacle to overcome with assisted reproduction, consider it an important health indicator deserving of thorough optimization.

The foundation of your fertility house depends as much on the quality of the support structure as it does on the primary building materials. Investing in complete structural enhancement rather than quick fixes often pays dividends in both reproductive outcomes and long-term health.

HIDDEN DAMAGE: INFECTIONS AND SCARRING IN THE FERTILITY STRUCTURE

In our home renovation metaphor, infections and scarring represent hidden damage within your fertility structure—similar to discovering mold behind walls or damaged connections in your home's plumbing and electrical systems. These issues may not be immediately visible but can significantly compromise the functionality of your reproductive system.

Just as a house with water damage or electrical shorts can't operate at peak performance, a reproductive system affected by past infections or accumulated scar tissue faces challenges that must be addressed before fertility can be optimized.

INFECTIONS: MICROBIAL INVADERS AND INFLAMMATORY RESPONSES
Understanding the Impact:
Infections in the reproductive system are like unwelcome microscopic invaders in your home's structure:

1. **Sexually Transmitted Infections (STIs):**
    - **Chlamydia:** Often silent, can travel up the reproductive tract and cause inflammation and scarring in fallopian tubes
    - **Gonorrhea:** May damage fallopian tubes and increase risk of ectopic pregnancy
    - **Mycoplasma/Ureaplasma:** Lesser-known infections that can affect sperm function and embryo implantation
    - **HPV (Human Papillomavirus):** Can affect cervical health and potentially impact fertility
    - **Herpes:** May affect conception timing and pregnancy management

2. **Reproductive Tract Infections:**
    - **Bacterial Vaginosis:** Alters vaginal microbiome, potentially affecting sperm survival
    - **Endometritis:** Inflammation of the uterine lining affecting implantation
    - **Chronic Endometrial Infection:** Persistent low-grade infection impairing receptivity
    - **Group B Streptococcus:** May persist after delivery and affect future pregnancies

3. **Procedural Infections:**
   o **Post-IUI Infections:** Inflammation following intrauterine insemination
   o **Post-Hysteroscopy/HSG:** Introduced bacteria during diagnostic procedures
   o **Chorioamnionitis:** Infection of fetal membranes during pregnancy that can leave residual inflammation

4. **Male Reproductive Infections:**
   o **Prostatitis:** Inflammation of the prostate affecting semen quality
   o **Epididymitis:** Infection in sperm transport structures
   o **Orchitis:** Testicular infection potentially affecting sperm production
   o **Seminal Vesiculitis:** Infection of seminal vesicles affecting semen composition

THE INFECTION-FERTILITY CONNECTION:
Reproductive infections impact fertility through multiple mechanisms:
1. **Structural Damage:**
   o Scarring and blockage of fallopian tubes
   o Adhesions in the pelvic cavity
   o Damage to sperm-producing tissues

2. **Inflammatory Environment:**
   o Altered pH affecting sperm survival
   o Hostile cervical mucus limiting sperm transport
   o Inflammation in the endometrium impairing implantation
   o Inflammatory cytokines affecting embryo development

3. **Microbial Imbalance:**
   - Disruption of healthy vaginal or seminal microbiome
   - Overgrowth of harmful bacteria
   - Displacement of beneficial flora that supports fertility

4. **Immune System Activation:**
   - Increased white blood cells attacking sperm
   - Development of anti-sperm antibodies
   - Chronic immune activation affecting implantation

DETECTION AND ASSESSMENT:

Identifying hidden infections often requires specialized investigation:

1. **Comprehensive Testing:**
   - Cervical/vaginal cultures for aerobic and anaerobic bacteria
   - Endometrial biopsy with microbiome analysis
   - Occasionally uterine culture may also be needed
   - Advanced STI screening including PCR testing
   - Semen cultures and white blood cell analysis
   - Immune marker testing (cytokines, NK cells)

2. **Specialized Diagnostics:**
   - EMMA test (Endometrial Microbiome Metagenomic Analysis)
   - ALICE test (Analysis of Infectious Chronic Endometritis)
   - ReceptivaDx test for endometritis and inflammation
   - Mycoplasma/Ureaplasma specific testing

SCARRING: STRUCTURAL LIMITATIONS FROM PAST DAMAGE

After my first IVF cycle transfers failed, I didn't want to jump right back into another cycle. I had researched and heard about Clear Passage therapy, and the closest destination was St. Louis, so off I went. I took a week away from the office—still podcasting and seeing patients virtually—to receive four days with twenty total hours of visceral manipulation.

I had a suspicion I had abdominal and pelvic scar tissue from my past surgeries and had previously suffered from SIBO, which I heard they could also help with. Clear Passage uses a non-surgical technique that involves essentially a specialized form of massage to break down abdominal adhesions. From their website:

> "The Wurn Technique® (WT) is a unique hands-on physio/physical therapy modality, developed over 30+ years by Belinda Wurn, PT, and Larry Wurn, LMT. It was initially created to decrease pain and increase function for Belinda, when adhesions from surgery and extensive radiation therapy left her unable to work due to debilitating chronic pain. Physicians said surgery would only make it worse because of the adhesions that inevitably form after surgery. They suggested she take drugs to mask the pain. Unwilling to endure a life of drugs and pain, Belinda and Larry began searching for a non-surgical cure. They took dozens of advanced courses in the U.S. and abroad, including study at a French medical school. They discovered that the body forms adhesions—powerful bonds similar to nylon curtains or ropes—to help injured tissues heal. Once healing has occurred, adhesions remain in the body, often binding tissues that were previously free to move naturally. When this happens,

pain and dysfunction are the natural result. As they developed their findings into a treatment, Belinda was able to return to a pain-free life. The WT was born from the Wurns' newfound knowledge."[2]

The technique is designed to deform and detach these tiny but powerful adhesions and return the body to normal, pain-free function. As a manual therapy, it works without the risks or side effects of surgery or drugs. What caught my attention was their track record—they had a higher success rate opening blocked fallopian tubes than surgery and similar outcomes as IVF, so I thought I'd give it a shot.

Boy, were they thorough. They did internal and external work on me, and I do think this was another crucial tool that ultimately led to my successful pregnancy. This was like Mercier therapy—a form of pelvic visceral manipulation that promotes organ mobility and restores optimal blood flow to the pelvic organs— but WAY more comprehensive.

COMMON SOURCES OF REPRODUCTIVE SCARRING:

Just as old water damage or electrical fires leave lasting structural impacts in a home, various events can create lasting scars in the reproductive system:

1. **Surgical Scarring:**
    - **C-section:** Creates uterine scar and potential abdominal adhesions
    - **Myomectomy:** Removal of fibroids leaving uterine scarring

---

[2] You can learn more about the Wurn Technique by visiting their website, https://clearpassage.com/our-story-the-clear-passage-approach/.

- **Laparoscopy:** Can create adhesions between pelvic structures
- **Appendectomy/Gallbladder Surgery:** Abdominal surgeries potentially affecting reproductive organ mobility
- **D&C Procedures:** Dilation and curettage potentially creating Asherman's syndrome (uterine scarring)

2. **Infection-Related Scarring:**
   - **PID (Pelvic Inflammatory Disease):** Leading cause of tubal factor infertility
   - **Endometritis:** Can lead to intrauterine adhesions
   - **Post-surgical Infections:** Worsening of adhesion formation

3. **Endometriosis-Related Scarring:**
   - Adhesions between organs limiting mobility
   - Scarring around ovaries affecting egg release
   - Distortion of pelvic anatomy

4. **Injury-Related Scarring:**
   - Physical trauma to reproductive organs
   - Accidents affecting pelvic structures
   - Sports injuries to testicular area

THE SCARRING-FERTILITY CONNECTION:

Scar tissue impacts fertility through several mechanisms:

1. **Mechanical Obstruction:**
   - Blocked fallopian tubes preventing egg transport

- Uterine adhesions (Asherman's syndrome) affecting implantation
- Cervical scarring limiting sperm entry

2. **Restricted Mobility:**
   - Adhesions limiting normal movement of reproductive organs
   - Restricted fallopian tube mobility affecting egg pickup
   - Limited uterine expansion during pregnancy

3. **Altered Blood Flow:**
   - Reduced circulation to scarred areas
   - Compromised endometrial vascularization
   - Diminished nutrient delivery to developing follicles

4. **Implantation Interference:**
   - Scarred endometrium with fewer receptors
   - Uneven endometrial growth
   - Impaired embryo attachment

DETECTION AND ASSESSMENT:

Identifying the extent of scarring requires various diagnostic approaches:

1. **Imaging Studies:**
   - Hysterosalpingogram (HSG) for tubal patency
   - Saline sonogram for intrauterine scarring
   - MRI for detailed tissue assessment
   - 3D ultrasound for uterine cavity evaluation

2. **Surgical Evaluation:**
    - Hysteroscopy for direct visualization of uterine cavity
    - Laparoscopy for pelvic adhesion assessment
    - Chromopertubation or hysterosalpingogram (HSG) to test tubal function

RESTORATION STRATEGIES: CLEARING INFECTIONS AND REMODELING SCARRED TISSUES

Infection Remediation (Conventional Approach):

The conventional approach to reproductive infections typically includes:

1. **Targeted Antibiotics:**
    - Specific antibiotic selection based on culture results
    - Often extended courses for chronic infections
    - Partner treatment when appropriate

2. **Procedural Interventions:**
    - Drainage of infected areas when needed
    - Removal of infected tissue
    - IUD removal if associated with infection

3. **Symptom Management:**
    - Anti-inflammatory medications
    - Pain management
    - Supportive care during treatment

Infection Remediation (Functional Approach):

A comprehensive functional approach includes:

1. **Targeted Antimicrobial Therapy:**
    - Conventional antibiotics when necessary
    - Biofilm-disrupting agents

- Botanical antimicrobials as appropriate:
  - Berberine for bacterial infections
  - Oregano oil for broad-spectrum support
  - Garlic for antifungal and antibacterial properties
  - Monolaurin for viral and bacterial issues

2. **Microbiome Restoration:**
   - Specific probiotic strains for reproductive health
   - Prebiotic support for beneficial bacteria
   - Vaginal microbiome optimization
   - Semen microbiome considerations

3. **Immune System Modulation:**
   - Reducing systemic inflammation
   - Supporting balanced immune response
   - Addressing autoimmune factors when present
   - Specialized supplements: NAC, quercetin, curcumin

4. **Mucosal Healing Support:**
   - L-glutamine for tissue repair
   - Zinc for epithelial integrity
   - Vitamin A for mucosal health
   - Collagen support for tissue strength

SCAR TISSUE MANAGEMENT (CONVENTIONAL APPROACH):

Conventional approaches to scarring typically involve:

1. **Surgical Interventions:**
   - Hysteroscopic adhesiolysis (which is a surgical procedure that involves the removal or separation of adhesions) for intrauterine scarring

- Laparoscopic adhesiolysis for pelvic adhesions
- Tubal reconstruction when possible
- Placement of barriers to prevent readhesion

2. **Mechanical Approaches:**
   - Placement of intrauterine balloons or stents
   - Cycling estrogen therapy after adhesiolysis
   - Physical therapy for external tissue scarring

3. **Bypass Methods:**
   - IVF to bypass tubal issues
   - Gestational carrier for severe uterine scarring
   - Donor sperm for severe male tract obstruction

SCAR TISSUE MANAGEMENT (FUNCTIONAL APPROACH):

A comprehensive approach to scar tissue management includes:

1. **Physical Manipulation Techniques:**
   - Specialized pelvic physical therapy
   - Visceral manipulation for organ mobility
   - Fascial release techniques like Mercier therapy
   - Wurn Technique with Clear Passage approach

2. **Anti-Fibrotic Supplementation:**
   - Systemic enzymes (serrapeptase, nattokinase) on empty stomach
   - Lumbrokinase for enhanced fibrinolytic activity
   - EGCG from green tea extract
   - Specialized fish oil formulations

3. **Anti-Inflammatory Support:**
   - Curcumin with enhanced bioavailability
   - Boswellia for specialized anti-inflammatory properties
   - SPMs (Specialized Pro-resolving Mediators)
   - Modified citrus pectin

4. **Circulation Enhancement:**
   - Nitric oxide precursors (L-arginine, L-citrulline)
   - Ginkgo biloba for microcirculation
   - Infrared light therapy
   - Specialized hydrotherapy approaches

5. **Collagen Remodeling Support:**
   - Vitamin C for proper collagen formation
   - Silicon for connective tissue health
   - Copper and manganese as enzyme cofactors
   - Specialized collagen peptides

> **Success Story:** Rachel, a 36-year-old teacher, had been trying to conceive for four years with unexplained infertility. She had undergone three IUI cycles and one round of IVF without success, despite having good embryo quality. During a comprehensive functional medicine assessment, and after reviewing her Creighton method charting (further explained at the end of Chapter 14 in the cervical mucus

monitoring section) that demonstrated tail-end brown bleeding, it was highly suspected that Rachel could have chronic, asymptomatic endometritis that hadn't been detected in her previous fertility workups. Testing also revealed an imbalanced vaginal microbiome with an overgrowth of certain bacteria.

She implemented a targeted protocol including specific antibiotic therapy followed by intensive probiotic treatment, vaginal microbiome restoration, and systemic enzyme therapy, and was referred for local Mercier therapy to address potential scar tissue.

Three months after completing treatment, Rachel conceived naturally during her first attempt. Her case highlights how "invisible" infections that don't cause obvious symptoms can significantly impact fertility and how addressing these hidden issues can restore natural conception abilities.

KEY TAKEAWAYS ON HIDDEN DAMAGE

When addressing fertility challenges, investigating for hidden damage from infections and scarring should be a standard consideration:

1. **Don't Overlook Past Events:**
    - Previous surgeries, even seemingly unrelated ones like appendectomy

- History of STIs, even those treated years ago
- Difficult deliveries or pregnancy complications
- Pelvic or abdominal injuries

2. **Connect Symptoms to Potential Hidden Damage:**
   - Unexplained pelvic pain
   - Pain with intercourse
   - Unusual discharge or recurrent infections
   - Changing menstrual patterns (brown bleeding)
   - Cyclical symptoms that worsen around periods

3. **Advocate for Comprehensive Testing:**
   - Standard fertility workups may miss chronic infections
   - Request specialized microbiome and inflammation testing
   - Consider immune system evaluation
   - Seek detailed imaging of reproductive structures

4. **Recognize the Interconnected Nature of Infections and Scarring:**
   - Infections often lead to scarring
   - Scarring can harbor persistent infections
   - Both create inflammatory environments
   - Addressing both simultaneously offers the best outcomes

The good news is that even longstanding hidden damage can often be significantly improved with the right approach. Just as a skilled renovation team can remediate old water damage and restore compromised structures in a home, targeted strategies can address infections and remodel scar tissue, creating a more receptive environment for conception and healthy pregnancy.

CIRCULATION COMPLICATIONS: BLOOD-CLOTTING DISORDERS AND REPRODUCTIVE SUCCESS

In our home renovation metaphor, blood-clotting disorders and methylation issues represent circulation complications in your fertility blueprint—similar to plumbing restrictions that prevent proper flow of water throughout your home. Just as restricted pipes can prevent water from reaching critical areas of your house, clotting disorders and impaired methylation pathways can disrupt crucial processes needed for successful reproduction, particularly affecting implantation and the developing placenta during pregnancy.

These circulation and metabolic pathway issues may not affect conception directly, but they can significantly impact implantation and pregnancy maintenance, leading to recurrent early pregnancy losses that might be mistaken for fertility problems. Of particular importance are MTHFR gene variants, which affect this critical metabolic process called methylation that impacts everything from detoxification to DNA repair to hormone metabolism.

THE PLUMBING PROBLEM: UNDERSTANDING CLOTTING DISORDERS

Key Circulation Complications:

Several blood-clotting disorders can affect reproductive success:
1. **Antiphospholipid Syndrome (APS):**
    - The most common acquired thrombophilia affecting pregnancy
    - Autoimmune condition where the body produces antibodies against its own phospholipids

- Three main antibodies tested: lupus anticoagulant, anticardiolipin antibodies, and anti-beta-2 glycoprotein I
- Associated with recurrent pregnancy loss, preeclampsia, intrauterine growth restriction, and placental insufficiency

2. **Inherited Thrombophilias:**
    - **Factor V Leiden:** Most common inherited thrombophilia; increases clotting tendency
    - **Prothrombin Gene Mutation (G20210A):** Causes elevated prothrombin levels
    - **MTHFR Gene Variants:** Important methylation pathway variants affecting folate metabolism:
        » **C677T Variant:** Reduces enzyme efficiency by 30–70% depending on homozygous/heterozygous status
        » **A1298C Variant:** Affects enzyme function and neurotransmitter metabolism
        » **Compound Heterozygosity:** Having both variants significantly impacts methylation
        » **Connection to Fertility:** May affect homocysteine levels, detoxification, neurotransmitter balance, and inflammatory responses
    - **Protein C and Protein S Deficiencies:** Reduced natural anticoagulants
    - **Antithrombin III Deficiency:** Lack of important clotting inhibitor

3. **Acquired Clotting Issues:**
    - **Elevated Homocysteine:** Can result from nutritional deficiencies or genetic factors
    - **Elevated Factor VIII:** Can occur in response to inflammation or stress
    - **Plasminogen Activator Inhibitor-1 (PAI-1) Elevation:** Reduces clot breakdown

HOW CLOTTING ISSUES AFFECT FERTILITY AND PREGNANCY:

Visualize your reproductive system's blood circulation as the plumbing in your home—when restrictions develop:

1. **Implantation Complications:**
    - Micro-clots in the uterine lining can prevent proper embryo attachment
    - Reduced blood flow to the endometrium affects receptivity
    - Inflammatory processes at the implantation site become dysregulated

2. **Early Placental Development Issues:**
    - Clotting in developing placental vessels restricts nutrient flow
    - Improper placentation due to compromised blood supply
    - Placental villi can't form properly with inadequate circulation

3. **Ongoing Pregnancy Challenges:**
   - Placental infarcts (areas of dead tissue) from clot formation
   - Reduced oxygen and nutrient delivery to the developing fetus
   - Increased risk of later pregnancy complications

WARNING SIGNS OF CIRCULATION PROBLEMS:

Just as water pressure issues signal plumbing problems in your home, several indicators suggest possible clotting disorders:

1. **Reproductive Warning Signs:**
   - Recurrent early pregnancy losses (especially after heartbeat detection)
   - Previous pregnancy complications (preeclampsia, HELLP syndrome, placental abruption)
   - Unexplained infertility with failed IVF implantation
   - Late-term pregnancy loss

2. **Personal and Family History Flags:**
   - Previous blood clots (DVT or pulmonary embolism)
   - Family history of clotting disorders or recurrent pregnancy loss
   - Autoimmune conditions (especially lupus, Sjögren's syndrome, or rheumatoid arthritis)
   - History of stroke or heart attack at young age (personal or family)
   - Migraine with aura
   - Livedo reticularis (lace-like purple skin discoloration)

3. **Coexisting Conditions:**
    - Other autoimmune disorders
    - History of abnormal blood tests
    - Unexplained inflammation
    - Chronic conditions with inflammatory components

INSPECTION METHODS: DIAGNOSING CLOTTING DISORDERS
Comprehensive Blood Flow Assessment:
Testing for clotting disorders typically involves:
1. **Antiphospholipid Antibody Panel:**
    - Lupus anticoagulant
    - Anticardiolipin antibodies (IgG, IgM, IgA)
    - Anti-beta-2 glycoprotein I antibodies (IgG, IgM, IgA)
    - Note: These tests should be performed twice, at least 12 weeks apart, for diagnosis

2. **Inherited Thrombophilia Testing:**
    - Factor V Leiden mutation
    - Prothrombin G20210A mutation
    - MTHFR gene mutations (C677T and A1298C)
    - Protein C and Protein S activity
    - Antithrombin III levels

3. **Additional Clotting Assessments:**
    - Homocysteine levels
    - Factor VIII activity
    - PAI-1 (plasminogen activator inhibitor-1) levels and 4G/5G genotyping
    - D-dimer (marker of active clotting)
    - Complete blood count with platelet evaluation

4. **Related Testing:**
   - Inflammatory markers (CRP, ESR, ferritin)
   - Comprehensive autoimmune panels
   - Vitamin D, B12, and folate levels

WHEN TESTING SHOULD BE CONSIDERED:
Clotting disorder evaluation is particularly important if you have:
- Two or more unexplained first-trimester losses
- One or more unexplained second-trimester losses
- History of preeclampsia, especially early-onset
- Severe intrauterine growth restriction in previous pregnancy
- History of placental abruption
- Unexplained stillbirth
- Family history of clotting disorders
- Multiple failed IVF cycles with good quality embryos (which was me!)
- Personal history of blood clots

FLOW RESTORATION: CONVENTIONAL AND FUNCTIONAL APPROACHES
Conventional Flow Restoration:
The standard medical approach focuses on anticoagulation:
1. **Anticoagulant Therapy:**
   - **Low-dose aspirin (81mg):** Often the first-line treatment
   - **Heparin injections:** Typically, low-molecular-weight heparin such as enoxaparin (Lovenox)
   - **Timing:** Usually started before conception or immediately upon pregnancy confirmation
   - **Duration:** Often continued until 6 weeks postpartum

2. **Additional Medications:**
   - Hydroxychloroquine for certain autoimmune components
   - Corticosteroids in specific circumstances
   - Intravenous immunoglobulin for refractory cases

3. **Specialized Monitoring:**
   - Extra ultrasounds for growth and placental function
   - Doppler studies of uterine and umbilical blood flow
   - More frequent prenatal visits

FUNCTIONAL FLOW ENHANCEMENT:

A comprehensive approach addresses both clotting factors and underlying causes:

1. **Natural Anticoagulant Support:**
   - **Omega-3 fatty acids:** 2–4g daily of EPA/DHA from quality fish oil
   - **Nattokinase:** Enzyme with fibrinolytic properties (avoid during active pregnancy)
   - **Systemic enzymes:** Specific formulations on empty stomach
   - **Ginger:** Moderate amounts for circulation enhancement
   - **Turmeric:** With enhanced bioavailability for anti-inflammatory effects

2. **Underlying Cause Remediation:**
   - **Autoimmune regulation:** LDN (low-dose naltrexone), specialized dietary approaches

- **Methylation support:** Active B vitamins (methylfolate, methylcobalamin)
- **Inflammation reduction:** SPMs, curcumin, boswellia, specialized diets
- **Gut health optimization:** Addressing intestinal permeability, microbiome support

3. **Nutritional Foundation:**
    - **Optimal B vitamin status:** Especially B6, folate, and B12
    - **Methylation support for MTHFR variants:**
        » Active forms of folate (L-methylfolate) rather than folic acid
        » Methylcobalamin (B12) and pyridoxal-5-phosphate (B6)
        » Supplemental riboflavin (B2), which supports MTHFR enzyme function
        » Betaine (TMG) as an alternative methyl donor
        » Choline to support methylation pathways
    - **Vitamin D optimization:** Typically, 50–80 ng/mL blood levels
    - **Antioxidant support:** Vitamin C, vitamin E, glutathione precursors
    - **Magnesium sufficiency:** 300–600mg daily of highly absorbable forms

4. **Circulation Enhancement:**
    - **Physical activity:** Appropriate movement to enhance blood flow

- **Hydration optimization:** Supporting blood viscosity
- **Hot/cold contrast therapies:** Improving vascular responsiveness
- **Specialized massage:** Enhancing peripheral circulation

> **Success Story:** Alana experienced three early pregnancy losses between 6–9 weeks, each time after seeing a heartbeat on ultrasound. Standard recurrent pregnancy loss workups found nothing concerning. When she sought a second opinion, comprehensive clotting panels revealed positive anticardiolipin antibodies and lupus anticoagulant, plus homozygous MTHFR C677T mutation with elevated homocysteine levels. She began a protocol combining low-dose aspirin, Lovenox injections upon confirmation of her next pregnancy, and functional support, including L-methylfolate (instead of standard folic acid), methylcobalamin B12, fish oil, vitamin D optimization, and an anti-inflammatory nutrition plan. She conceived again within two months and maintained the pregnancy with close monitoring, delivering a healthy baby girl at 38 weeks. For her subsequent pregnancy two years later, she followed the same protocol with similar success.

THE BLOOD FLOW-FERTILITY CONNECTION: ENSURING CRITICAL CIRCULATION

The connection between blood-clotting disorders and reproductive success illustrates an important principle: fertility isn't just about producing eggs and sperm or having open fallopian tubes—it's also about creating and maintaining the perfect environment for implantation and development.

KEY CONSIDERATIONS FOR OPTIMIZING CIRCULATION:

1. **Proactive Testing Is Crucial:**
   - Don't wait for multiple losses to investigate clotting disorders
   - Consider testing before attempting pregnancy if you have risk factors
   - Ensure complete testing rather than limited panels
   - Include MTHFR genetic testing, especially for those with:
     » Family history of cardiovascular disease
     » History of recurrent pregnancy loss
     » Personal or family history of blood clots
     » Autoimmune conditions
     » Unexplained infertility
   - Repeat positive tests to confirm results

2. **Treatment Should Begin Early:**
   - For confirmed clotting disorders, treatment should ideally start before conception
   - At minimum, treatment should begin immediately upon pregnancy confirmation
   - Continuation through the postpartum period is often necessary

3. **Combination Approaches Often Work Best:**
   - Medical anticoagulation provides immediate protection
   - Functional approaches address underlying causes
   - Nutritional support enhances medication effectiveness
   - Lifestyle modifications improve overall circulation

4. **Monitoring Makes a Difference:**
   - Regular ultrasounds to assess placental development
   - Specialized blood flow studies when indicated
   - Ongoing assessment of clotting parameters
   - Adjustment of protocols as pregnancy progresses

UNDERSTANDING MTHFR'S IMPACT ON FERTILITY:

MTHFR variants deserve special attention in fertility discussions because they affect much more than just clotting:

1. **Methylation's Critical Role:**
   - Methylation affects over 200 processes in the body
   - These processes impact egg quality, sperm health, hormone balance, and detoxification
   - Proper methylation is necessary for gene expression and DNA repair

2. **Beyond Homocysteine:**
   - While elevated homocysteine is one concern with MTHFR variants, the effects extend further
   - Impaired methylation affects neurotransmitter balance (potentially worsening stress responses)
   - Detoxification capacity is reduced, allowing more reproductive toxins to accumulate
   - Cellular energy production may be compromised

3. **MTHFR and Recurrent Pregnancy Loss:**
   o Studies show certain MTHFR variants increase miscarriage risk 2–3 fold
   o The effect is more pronounced in women with homozygous C677T variant
   o The mechanism involves both potential clotting issues and impaired cellular processes

4. **Practical Management:**
   o Avoid synthetic folic acid, which can block folate receptors in those with variants
   o Use active folate forms (L-methylfolate) in prenatal vitamins
   o Support the entire methylation cycle with cofactors
   o Monitor homocysteine levels as a functional marker of methylation status

For many women with unexplained recurrent pregnancy loss or failed implantation, addressing previously undetected clotting disorders and methylation issues can be the missing piece that allows successful pregnancy. Unlike many other fertility challenges that affect conception, these factors primarily impact the crucial early weeks after conception has already occurred—making them both particularly heartbreaking and often highly treatable with proper identification.

In our home renovation metaphor, ensuring proper "plumbing flow" throughout your reproductive system may be the critical factor that allows your fertility blueprint to finally succeed—not by changing the blueprint itself, but by ensuring that all systems can function as designed without restriction.

MY PERSONAL RENOVATION JOURNEY: WHEN HIDDEN DAMAGE MEETS CIRCULATION COMPLICATIONS

After helping countless patients overcome their fertility challenges, I faced my own complex renovation project that taught me firsthand how hidden damage and circulation issues can sabotage even the most promising fertility blueprints. My story illustrates why a comprehensive approach is so crucial, and why persistence in finding the root cause can make all the difference.

Despite having what appeared to be excellent building materials—high-quality eggs that created numerous euploid (chromosomally normal) embryos through IVF—my body wasn't able to successfully implant and maintain a pregnancy. As one resident said after my second egg retrieval: "If you don't get pregnant, if these don't take, you need to play the lottery." The statistics were in my favor—with three euploid embryos, success rates should have been around 97%. Yet transfer after transfer failed.

This told me something profound: we had great eggs, sperm, and embryos, but something else was preventing successful implantation. My instincts as both a provider and a patient led me to suspect my uterine environment.

Uncovering the Hidden Damage

Early in my journey, I had requested a uterine biopsy because I suspected that a previous chorioamnionitis (uterine infection from labor) might be causing implantation failure. The standard blind biopsy came back normal, and I temporarily laid that hypothesis to rest. But after a year of continued failures, including an early loss during my second IVF cycle, I knew something still wasn't right.

Rather than continue transferring valuable euploid embryos into a potentially compromised environment, I made an unusual request:

another surgery. As I told my doctor, "There is a reason this isn't working. Rather than keep wasting euploid embryos, let's look into my uterus or get a surrogate."

This persistence paid off. Unlike the blind biopsies done previously, during surgery the doctor could visually identify areas of concern. The upper pole of my uterus—precisely where they had been deploying all those embryos—showed significant inflammation, and I had endometritis. This confirmed my long-held suspicion that the previous chorioamnionitis had left lasting damage, creating an inhospitable environment for embryo implantation.

I firmly believe that I never actually needed IVF. What I needed was proper diagnosis and treatment of the underlying uterine inflammation and damage.

Addressing Circulation Complications
My research had also pointed to another potential issue: blood-clotting disorders. Knowing I had MTHFR genetic variants, I decided to test myself for antiphospholipid syndrome. Just as I had been surprised to discover I had celiac disease through self-testing (as I shared in *Your Longevity Blueprint*), I was shocked when some of the blood tests came back positive for antiphospholipid antibodies.

Further testing at the University of Iowa Hospitals and Clinics (UIHC) showed that while I didn't meet all the clinical criteria for full antiphospholipid syndrome (I hadn't had a miscarriage beyond ten weeks or experienced a blood clot), my history of failed euploid transfers combined with the positive blood work was enough to warrant treatment with a blood-thinning medication, Lovenox. Though I wasn't thrilled about taking injections, my determination to have a successful pregnancy outweighed any hesitation.

The Complete Renovation Approach

Following surgery to address the inflammation and endometritis, I was treated with antibiotics to clear any lingering infection. To ensure the surgical work didn't lead to scarring and to maintain tissue mobility, I underwent Mercier Therapy. For my next embryo transfer, I was on both blood thinners aspirin and Lovenox to prevent clotting issues, and I continued progesterone support—of course, along with the prenatal vitamin with methylfolate and methylcobalamin and fish oil. This comprehensive approach—addressing both the hidden damage in my uterus and the circulation issues—finally led to success. After seven transfers, eight embryos total, this pregnancy lasted!

Throughout my pregnancy, I followed the Pope Paul VI Institute progesterone protocol and continued progesterone injections to support the pregnancy. I wasn't taking any chances after such a long journey.

THE BLUEPRINT LESSON

My personal story reveals a crucial truth about fertility challenges: sometimes it's not about the quality of your building materials (eggs and sperm) but about creating the right environment for them to thrive. We needed to both address the inflamed, possibly infected uterine environment and ensure proper blood flow wasn't being compromised by clotting factors.

Many women go through multiple rounds of fertility treatments without anyone looking deeper into these two critical factors. My medical knowledge allowed me to advocate for the testing and treatments I needed, but I share my story so you don't have to struggle through the same learning process.

If you're facing unexplained implantation failure or pregnancy loss—especially with good-quality embryos—consider whether hidden inflammation/infection or blood-clotting disorders might be affecting your fertility blueprint. These issues can be addressed with the right approach, potentially saving you years of heartache and unnecessary procedures.

Like any thorough home renovation, sometimes you need to look behind the walls and check the plumbing before you can create a space where new life can flourish.

CHAPTER 14

INTEGRATION CHALLENGES—COMPREHENSIVE INFERTILITY ASSESSMENT

INFERTILITY: BLUEPRINT INTEGRATION CHALLENGES

In our home renovation metaphor, comprehensive infertility represents the ultimate blueprint integration challenge—a situation where multiple systems and structures must be carefully assessed and harmonized to create a functional whole. Just as a full home renovation requires coordinating electrical, plumbing, foundation, and aesthetic elements into a cohesive design, addressing complex fertility challenges demands a systematic approach that integrates all aspects of reproductive health.

When multiple factors contribute to fertility difficulties, success depends not just on addressing individual issues but on ensuring all systems work together seamlessly.

FULL PROPERTY INSPECTION: COMPREHENSIVE FERTILITY WORKUP
THE COMPLETE ASSESSMENT APPROACH:

A thorough fertility evaluation is like a comprehensive home inspection that leaves no system unchecked:

1. **Female Structural Assessment:**
   - Transvaginal ultrasound to evaluate uterus, ovaries, and follicles
   - Hysterosalpingogram (HSG) or sonohysterogram to assess fallopian tube patency and uterine cavity
   - Hysteroscopy when indicated for direct visualization of the uterine cavity
   - MRI for specific structural concerns

2. **Male Structural Evaluation:**
   - Semen analysis (ideally repeated 2–3 times)
   - Scrotal ultrasound when indicated
   - Advanced sperm function testing when appropriate
   - Physical examination for varicocele or other abnormalities

3. **Hormonal System Analysis:**
   - **Female Hormones:**
     » Day 3 FSH, LH, estradiol
     » AMH (anti-Müllerian hormone) for ovarian reserve
     » Progesterone (day 21, or 7 days post-ovulation)
     » Thyroid panel (TSH, free T3, free T4, TPO antibodies)
     » Androgens (testosterone, DHEA-S)
     » Prolactin

- **Male Hormones:**
  - Testosterone (total and free)
  - FSH and LH
  - Estradiol
  - Thyroid function
  - Prolactin when indicated

4. **Immune System Investigation:**
   - Antiphospholipid antibodies
   - Thyroid antibodies
   - Antisperm antibodies when indicated
   - Natural killer cell activity for recurrent losses
   - Reproductive immunophenotype

5. **Genetic Blueprint Review:**
   - Karyotyping when indicated
   - MTHFR and other thrombophilia testing
   - Carrier screening for hereditary conditions
   - Sperm DNA fragmentation
   - Specialized genetic panels based on history

6. **Metabolic Foundation Inspection:**
   - Glucose regulation (fasting glucose, insulin, HbA1c)
   - Inflammatory markers (CRP, homocysteine)
   - Nutritional status assessment
   - Oxidative stress markers when available

7. **Environmental Influence Evaluation:**
   - Toxin exposure history
   - Occupational hazards assessment

- Home environment review
- Water and food quality considerations

8. **Gut Foundation Check:**
   - Food sensitivity testing
   - Comprehensive stool profile

THE INTEGRATION CHALLENGE:
The true complexity in fertility assessment isn't just identifying individual issues but understanding how they interact:

- Hormonal imbalances may affect structural function
- Structural issues can trigger immune responses
- Genetic factors may influence hormonal systems
- Environmental factors can impact all other systems

This intricate web of interactions means that addressing just one component—even successfully—may not resolve fertility challenges if other factors remain unaddressed.

MATERIALS ASSESSMENT: EGG QUALITY, SPERM QUALITY, AND NURTURING ENVIRONMENT

The Essential Building Materials:
Just as a home renovation requires quality materials to succeed, reproduction depends on three fundamental components:

1. **Egg Quality Assessment:**
   - **Direct Measures:**
     » Follicle size and appearance on ultrasound
     » Number of eggs retrieved in IVF
     » Egg appearance and maturity in the lab

- » Fertilization rates and embryo development

- **Indirect Indicators:**
  - » Age (the strongest predictor of egg quality)
  - » AMH and antral follicle count (quantity indicators)
  - » FSH levels (elevated levels suggest diminished quality)
  - » Previous pregnancy outcomes

- **Functional Factors Affecting Quality:**
  - » Mitochondrial function (cellular energy production)
  - » Chromosomal stability
  - » Cytoplasmic maturity
  - » Oxidative stress levels
  - » Telomere length

2. **Sperm Quality Evaluation:**
   - **Standard Parameters:**
     - » Count (concentration of sperm)
     - » Motility (movement capacity)
     - » Morphology (shape and structure)
     - » Volume and pH of semen

   - **Advanced Assessments:**
     - » DNA fragmentation index (DFI)
     - » Oxidative stress testing
     - » Capacitation potential
     - » Hyaluronan binding assay
     - » Acrosome reaction testing

- **Contributing Factors:**
  - Age (less impactful than female age but still significant)
  - Environmental exposures
  - Varicocele presence
  - Lifestyle factors (heat, toxins, nutrition)
  - Abstinence duration

3. **Nurturing Environment Examination:**
   - **Uterine Factors:**
     - Endometrial thickness and pattern
     - Subendometrial blood flow
     - Presence of polyps, fibroids, or adhesions
     - Endometrial receptivity markers when available

   - **Cervical Factors:**
     - Cervical mucus quality and quantity
     - Cervical stenosis or abnormalities
     - Post-coital testing when indicated

   - **Fallopian Tube Assessment:**
     - Patency (openness)
     - Fimbrial health and mobility
     - Presence of adhesions or hydrosalpinx

   - **Immunological Environment:**
     - Cytokine balance
     - Presence of anti-embryo antibodies
     - Natural killer cell activity
     - HLA compatibility issues

MATERIAL QUALITY OPTIMIZATION:

When material quality issues are identified, targeted approaches can help:

1. **Egg Quality Enhancement (can be tailored based on nutrient testing):**
    - CoQ10 supplementation (typically 600mg daily)
    - Antioxidant protocols (NAC, melatonin, vitamin E, etc.)
    - Mitochondrial support (PQQ, resveratrol)
    - Anti-inflammatory nutrition
    - Stress reduction (cortisol management)
    - Appropriate exercise balance

2. **Sperm Quality Improvement (can be tailored based on nutrient testing):**
    - Antioxidant supplementation (especially zinc, selenium)
    - Heat reduction strategies
    - Toxin elimination
    - L-carnitine and acetyl-L-carnitine
    - Lifestyle optimization (alcohol reduction, smoking cessation)
    - Varicocele repair when indicated

3. **Nurturing Environment Enhancement:**
    - Hormone balance optimization
    - Endometrial scratch or PRP when appropriate
    - Immunomodulation for immune issues
    - Infection clearance, if present
    - Structural correction (polyp/fibroid removal)
    - Blood flow enhancement strategies

FUNCTIONAL CUSTOM BUILDING: INTEGRATING NATURAL APPROACHES

Timing Is Everything

For couples trying to conceive, the timing of intercourse plays a crucial role in success rates. The optimal approach is to "front-load" sexual activity in the days leading up to ovulation, rather than waiting until ovulation occurs. This strategy takes advantage of sperm's ability to survive in the female reproductive tract for several days while waiting for the egg's release.

Most men require 1–2 days to replenish their sperm supply to optimal levels, making intercourse every other day during the fertile window more effective than daily attempts. This schedule ensures both adequate sperm count and proper timing. The statistics bear this out: approximately 80% of pregnancies conceived at home occur when intercourse happens before ovulation, not during or after it.

This front-loading approach maximizes the chances that healthy, viable sperm are already positioned and waiting when the egg is released, rather than racing against time after ovulation has already begun. Since the egg remains viable for only 12–24 hours after ovulation, having sperm already present in the reproductive tract significantly improves the odds of successful fertilization during this narrow window of opportunity.

NATURAL CONSTRUCTION TIMELINE: TRACKING AND OPTIMIZING YOUR CYCLE

Understanding your body's natural rhythms provides crucial information:
1. **Basal Body Temperature (BBT) Charting:**
    - **The Process:** Taking temperature immediately upon waking

- **Pattern Recognition:** Identifying pre-ovulatory lower temperatures and post-ovulatory rise
- **Fertility Insights:**
  - Confirming ovulation is occurring
  - Determining the timing of ovulation
  - Assessing luteal phase length and adequacy
  - Identifying potential hormonal imbalances

- **Optimization Strategies:**
  - Digital thermometers with memory function
  - Temperature-tracking apps
  - Consistent timing for readings
  - Interpreting patterns rather than single readings

2. **Ovulation Predictor Kits (OPKs):**
   - **Standard OPKs:** Detect LH surge preceding ovulation
   - **Advanced Monitors:** Track multiple hormones (estrogen and LH)
   - **Practical Application:**
     - Begin testing based on shortest cycle length
     - Test same time daily (afternoon often best)
     - Continue until positive, then for one day after
     - Combine with other tracking methods

3. **Cycle Syncing Approaches:**
   - Aligning nutrition with cycle phases
   - Adjusting exercise intensity based on hormonal fluctuations
   - Timing supplements strategically throughout cycle
   - Modifying work and social demands when possible

MATERIAL QUALITY ASSESSMENT: CERVICAL MUCUS MONITORING

Cervical mucus provides a visible window into fertility status:

1. **Understanding Cervical Mucus Patterns:**
    - **Menstruation Phase:** Little to no mucus
    - **Post-Menstrual Phase:** Dry or sticky, non-fertile mucus
    - **Pre-Ovulatory Phase:** Increasing wetness, creamier texture
    - **Ovulatory Phase:** Clear, stretchy, slippery "egg white" mucus (peak fertility)
    - **Post-Ovulatory Phase:** Return to sticky or dry pattern

2. **Tracking Techniques:**
    - External observation with toilet paper
    - Manual collection with clean fingers
    - Daily consistency notation in fertility app
    - Classification systems (Billings or Creighton methods)

3. **Mucus Quality Enhancement:**
    - Hydration optimization (typically 80+ ounces of water daily)
    - Guaifenesin during fertile window
    - N-Acetyl Cysteine, also known as NAC
    - L-arginine supplementation
    - Elimination of antihistamines near ovulation
    - Avoiding lubricants that harm sperm

4. **Practical Application in Fertility Planning:**
    - Identifying the beginning of the fertile window
    - Recognizing peak fertility day(s)

- Timing intercourse with optimal mucus
- Assessing hormonal health through mucus patterns

ARCHITECTURAL PLANNING: FERTILITY AWARENESS METHODS

Structured natural family planning approaches offer systematic fertility tracking:

1. **The Creighton Model:**
   - **Foundation:** Standardized system of cervical mucus observation
   - **Unique Features:**
     - Standardized recordings with stamps/stickers
     - Trained practitioner guidance
     - Integration with NaProTECHNOLOGY medical treatment
     - Identification of abnormal bleeding patterns
   - **Fertility Applications:**
     - Precise identification of fertile window
     - Detection of hormonal abnormalities
     - Monitoring effects of treatments
     - Tracking cycle improvements over time

2. **Symptothermal Methods:**
   - **Combination Approach:** Using multiple fertility signs together
   - **Signs Monitored:**
     - Basal body temperature
     - Cervical mucus changes
     - Cervical position and firmness

- » Secondary symptoms (mittelschmerz, breast tenderness)

  o **Benefits for Fertility Challenges:**
    - » More precise window identification
    - » Cross-checking between signs
    - » Earlier detection of imbalances
    - » Better timing for treatment interventions

3. **Modern Fertility Awareness Technology:**
   - o Advanced tracking apps with algorithm predictions
   - o Wearable devices monitoring temperature patterns
   - o Hormone test integration with digital tracking
   - o AI analysis of personal patterns

> **Success Story:** After two years of unexplained infertility and one failed IUI cycle, Maya and David decided to take an integrative approach. While working with a reproductive endocrinologist, they also consulted a functional medicine practitioner who specialized in fertility. Comprehensive testing revealed subtle issues: borderline hypothyroidism, mild endometriosis, and moderate sperm DNA fragmentation—none severe enough alone to prevent pregnancy, but collectively creating significant challenges.

Their integrative plan included three months of preparation (CoQ10 for both partners, an anti-inflammatory diet, thyroid optimization, and specific supplementation) while learning the Creighton Model for precise cycle tracking. When they proceeded with their next IUI, they timed it based on Maya's peak fertility signs rather than a standard protocol day. This combined approach—conventional treatment enhanced with functional medicine and fertility awareness—resulted in a successful pregnancy on their next attempt.

CHAPTER 15

MEDICAL CONSTRUCTION METHODS

CONVENTIONAL CONSTRUCTION METHODS: WHEN TO CONSIDER MEDICAL INTERVENTION

Prefabricated Solutions: Ovulation Induction and IUI

For mild to moderate fertility challenges, these approaches offer targeted interventions:

1. **Ovulation Induction Medications:**
    - **Clomiphene Citrate (Clomid):** Stimulates FSH release by blocking estrogen receptors
    - **Letrozole (Femara):** Works by temporarily lowering estrogen to trigger FSH increase
    - **Gonadotropins:** Direct stimulation with FSH/LH injections
    - **Timing in Treatment:** Typically used for 3–6 cycles before moving to more advanced interventions

2. **Intrauterine Insemination (IUI):**
   - **The Process:** Concentrated sperm placed directly into uterus, bypassing cervical barriers
   - **Best Candidates:**
     » Mild male factor infertility
     » Cervical factor issues
     » Unexplained infertility
     » Sexual function difficulties
     » Single women

   - **Success Factors:**
     » Woman's age (significantly higher success under 35)
     » Total motile sperm count (ideally >10 million)
     » Presence of at least one open fallopian tube
     » Timing with ovulation

3. **Combined Approaches:**
   - Medication + timed intercourse
   - Medication + IUI (most common approach)
   - Medication + trigger shot + IUI (most precisely timed approach)

CHAPTER 16

ADVANCED MEDICAL INTERVENTIONS

COMPLETE REBUILD: IN VITRO FERTILIZATION (IVF)

When simpler approaches aren't sufficient, IVF represents a comprehensive reconstruction. However, just as a complete home rebuild still requires quality materials and proper preparation, IVF outcomes depend significantly on the health of eggs, sperm, and the reproductive environment—areas where functional medicine can make a profound difference.

1. **The Full IVF Process:**
    - **Ovarian Stimulation:** Medications to develop multiple follicles
    - **Monitoring:** Serial ultrasounds and blood tests to track response
    - **Trigger Shot:** Final maturation of eggs
    - **Egg Retrieval:** Surgical collection of eggs
    - **Fertilization:** Combining eggs and sperm in laboratory

- **Embryo Culture:** Growing embryos for 3–5 days
- **Embryo Transfer:** Placement of embryo(s) into uterus
- **Luteal Support:** Hormones to maintain early pregnancy

2. **Advanced IVF Technologies:**
   - **ICSI (Intracytoplasmic Sperm Injection):** Direct injection of sperm into egg
   - **Assisted Hatching:** Creating small opening in embryo's outer shell
   - **PGT (Preimplantation Genetic Testing):** Screening embryos for genetic issues
   - **ERA (Endometrial Receptivity Analysis):** Identifying optimal transfer window
   - **Embryo Freezing:** Preserving embryos for future use

3. **Functional Medicine Enhancement of IVF Outcomes:**
   - **Pre-IVF Optimization Period:** Typically 3–4 months of preparation before starting IVF
   - **Comprehensive Nutritional Analysis:**
     » Micronutrient testing to identify specific deficiencies
     » Customized supplementation based on individual needs
     » Focus on key fertility nutrients: CoQ10, Vitamin D, omega-3s, antioxidants
     » Optimization of protein intake (minimum 80–100g daily during IVF)

- Anti-Inflammatory Protocol:
  - Elimination of pro-inflammatory foods (gluten, dairy, sugar, processed foods)
  - Emphasis on anti-inflammatory foods (fatty fish, berries, leafy greens, olive oil)
  - Strategic use of anti-inflammatory supplements (curcumin, resveratrol, omega-3s)
  - Reduction of environmental inflammatory triggers

- Mitochondrial Support:
  - High-dose CoQ10 (600–800mg daily) for improved cellular energy
  - PQQ to increase mitochondrial numbers
  - L-carnitine for fatty acid transport into mitochondria
  - NAC and alpha-lipoic acid for antioxidant protection

- Stress Reduction Protocol:
  - Cortisol management through mind-body practices
  - Targeted adaptogenic herbs during IVF preparation
  - Strategic sleep optimization
  - Specific exercise recommendations during stimulation

- Detoxification Support:
  - Liver support throughout the process
  - Appropriate detoxification before beginning medications

» Environmental toxin reduction
» Clean beauty and home products during treatment

4. **Measurable Impacts of Functional Approaches on IVF Outcomes:**
    o Increased number of mature eggs retrieved
    o Improved fertilization rates
    o Higher quality embryos with better morphology
    o Increased blastocyst formation rates
    o Higher implantation rates
    o Reduced chemical pregnancy rate
    o Better pregnancy maintenance

5. **IVF Success Factors:**
    o Woman's age (primary determinant)
    o Embryo quality (significantly impacted by functional approaches)
    o Uterine receptivity (improved through inflammation reduction)
    o Clinic-specific protocols
    o Underlying fertility diagnosis
    o Pre-IVF preparation quality

6. **When IVF Is Most Indicated:**
    o Tubal factor infertility
    o Severe male factor
    o Diminished ovarian reserve
    o Genetic concerns requiring PGT

- Failed simpler treatments
- Advanced reproductive age

7. **Clinical Evidence for Functional Enhancement:**
    - Research shows CoQ10 supplementation increases egg yields by 20–30%
    - Mediterranean diet adherence improves successful implantation rates
    - Vitamin D sufficiency correlates with 33% higher live birth rates
    - Antioxidant protocols improve embryo quality markers
    - Stress reduction techniques show measurable benefits in IVF outcomes

FAITH AND FERTILITY: A PERSONAL JOURNEY

The decision to pursue IVF often brings unexpected spiritual considerations that many couples never anticipated facing. For those with strong faith backgrounds, the technology can initially feel like overstepping divine boundaries—a sense of "playing God" with the creation of life. This internal conflict is deeply personal and completely understandable.

As someone who never imagined considering IVF, I found myself grappling with these very questions when faced with the reality of potential infertility. The journey forced me to reexamine my understanding of divine providence and medical intervention. I was reminded of the parable of the man in the flood who refused multiple rescue attempts, saying, "I'm waiting for God to save me," only to discover in the end that God had sent him exactly the help he needed through human hands.

This perspective transformed how I viewed fertility treatments. Just as millions of people rely on conventional medicine for mood disorders, digestive issues, chronic pain, and countless other conditions, fertility medicine becomes another tool in the medical arsenal. We don't question whether God approves of insulin for diabetics or chemotherapy for cancer patients—these are viewed as blessings of medical knowledge and skill.

Ultimately, regardless of the method—natural conception, medication assistance, or advanced reproductive technology—only God creates life. The spark that transforms cells into a living being remains a divine mystery that no human technology can truly replicate or control. IVF and other fertility treatments simply provide the opportunity; the miracle of life itself remains firmly in higher hands. For many couples, these medical tools become answered prayers, allowing families to form that might not otherwise exist.

MY IVF STORY: THE POWER OF ANTIOXIDANTS IN CREATING QUALITY EMBRYOS

Before I share my experience, I want to explain some terminology for those who haven't gone through IVF or are considering it. What you're hoping for is creating euploid embryos—those that have the correct number of chromosomes, 46 (23 pairs). This is considered genetically normal and is the most desirable type of embryo in assisted reproductive technologies like IVF. Bottom line: euploid embryos have a significantly better chance of implanting in the uterus and resulting in a live birth compared to aneuploid (abnormal chromosome number) embryos.

Prior to conceiving Michael, I completed two IVF cycles that told a remarkable story about the power of optimization between attempts.

FIRST IVF CYCLE: GOOD NUMBERS, STANDARD RESULTS

With my first cycle, 24 eggs were harvested. Only 10 fertilized, and 5 turned into blastocysts (day-5 embryos). We transferred 2 embryos fresh, while the remaining 3 were sent for genetic testing. Of those tested, only 1 came back euploid.

Given my age, having 1 euploid embryo out of 3 tested met the expected 33% average, so in this round, I had either a 33% euploid rate or possibly higher, if one of the first 2 transferred embryos was also euploid. However, I'll never know since they weren't tested.

SECOND IVF CYCLE: DRAMATIC IMPROVEMENT

My second cycle was completely different. I had the same number of eggs harvested—24—but the looks on the residents' faces showed these eggs just appeared higher quality from the start. This time, 16 eggs fertilized (versus 10 in the first cycle), and 9 turned into blastocysts (versus 5 in the first cycle).

But here's where it gets interesting: this round produced 5 euploid embryos and 1 mosaic embryo (which can sometimes be transferred depending on the clinic's protocols). Depending on how you calculate it, either 4/9 = 44% or 5/9 = 56% were transferable quality—far above the 33% average for my age group.

These statistics were incredible. As reproductive endocrinologists say, "It's a numbers game." I had the numbers—boy oh boy, for my age I had incredible numbers.

WHAT MADE THE DIFFERENCE?

I will never know for certain why the second cycle produced so many more high-quality euploid embryos, but I can identify two major differences between cycles:

1. My husband's health optimization: Eric had his gallbladder removed between retrievals and focused on rebuilding his nutritional status and overall health
2. My intensive antioxidant protocol: I significantly increased my antioxidant intake, specifically adding C60 (Carbon 60) to my regimen

THE NUMBERS GAME REALITY

With three euploid embryos, a woman has a high chance of achieving pregnancy through IVF, with success rates reported to be around 97%. But this isn't always the case—many women have a very difficult time creating euploid embryos, which is heartbreaking when you understand that embryo quality is often the determining factor in IVF success.

MY STRONG BELIEF: OXIDATIVE STRESS IS THE KEY

It is my firm belief that mitigating oxidative stress was the secret to creating so many euploid embryos. You can do this through everything mentioned in this book—the nutrition protocols, environmental cleanup, stress reduction, and targeted supplementation—plus strategic antioxidant support.

You don't have to take my word for it. In Dr. Casey Means' 2024 book *Good Energy*, she also heavily emphasizes the importance of reducing oxidative stress for improving fertility outcomes, regardless of diagnosis or medical label.

The eggs retrieved in my second cycle had been developing for approximately 100 days—the entire time I was implementing intensive antioxidant protocols. Those eggs were literally bathed in antioxidant protection during their final maturation phase, and the results speak for themselves.

THE ANTIOXIDANT ADVANTAGE

I truly believe that antioxidants made the difference for me, and they can help you too—whether you're trying to conceive naturally or preparing for IVF. The protocols in this book are designed to create the optimal internal environment for egg and sperm development, reducing the oxidative damage that can lead to chromosomal abnormalities.

This is why the preparation phase is so crucial. The eggs you ovulate this month began their development 100 days ago. The eggs you'll ovulate three months from now are developing right now, and you have the power to influence their quality through the choices you make today.

THE POWER OF INTEGRATION: COMBINING APPROACHES FOR OPTIMAL RESULTS

The most effective approach to complex fertility challenges often involves thoughtful integration of conventional and functional methods:

1. **Staged Treatment Approach:**
    - Beginning with least invasive, most natural approaches
    - Adding targeted conventional interventions as needed
    - Advancing to more comprehensive treatments when indicated
    - Maintaining core functional supports throughout

2. **Enhancing Conventional Treatments:**
    - Optimizing natural fertility before beginning medical treatments
    - Supporting egg and sperm quality during medication cycles
    - Using fertility awareness to perfect medical treatment timing

- Addressing underlying factors even during advanced treatments

3. **Personalized Integration Strategy:**
   - Considering age and time constraints
   - Respecting personal preferences and values
   - Acknowledging financial considerations
   - Balancing emotional well-being with medical urgency

4. **Communication Between Approaches:**
   - Keeping all healthcare providers informed
   - Understanding potential interactions
   - Documenting responses to all interventions
   - Creating a coordinated care timeline

The blueprint integration challenge of infertility is perhaps the most complex renovation project your body can face—but with thorough assessment, quality materials, appropriate construction methods, and attention to natural rhythms, even the most challenging fertility blueprints can often lead to successful outcomes.

Whether you ultimately conceive through completely natural means, with minimal assistance, or through advanced reproductive technology, the fundamental principles remain the same: **creating the optimal conditions for life to begin and flourish, just as a well-executed renovation creates the perfect environment for a house to become a home.**

YOUR LONGEVITY BLUEPRINT (LB) NUTRACEUTICAL PRODUCTS:

Note: Throughout this book, I share Your Longevity Blueprint nutraceutical products, which we use at the Integrative Health and Hormone Clinic. Our brand is evidence-based—we've created formulations specifically designed for fertility optimization that work. We maintain the highest standards for our raw materials and use only the most therapeutic potencies needed to support reproductive health. Learn more at yourlongevityblueprint.com.

Here are my favorite LB products to address needs mentioned in this section:

- Adrenal Calm
- Alpha Lipoic Acid
- Antioxidant Support
- Complete Turmeric Complex
- CoQ10
- DHEA
- DIM
- Enzyme Support
- GLP Fiber Complex
- GI Support
- Gut shield
- Herbal Adrenal Complex
- Inositol Complex
- L-Theanine
- Magnesium Chelate
- Methyl B complex
- Metabolism Support
- Mitochondrial Complex
- NAC
- NeuroSupport Mag
- Omega3s (fish oil)
- SL Methyl Bs
- Vitamin D3
- Vitamin D3 with K2 liquid and capsule
- Zinc Chelate

You can download product data sheets with details about each of these products at yourlongevityblueprint.com, and use the code "fertility" for 10% off.

Advanced Medical Interventions

SECTION V

DIY FERTILITY IMPROVEMENTS—OPTIMIZING YOUR REPRODUCTIVE HOME

CHAPTER 17

STRUCTURAL FOUNDATION WORK

While professional help is often needed for complex fertility challenges, there's much you can do on your own to improve your reproductive health. Just as a homeowner can make significant improvements to their property before calling in specialized contractors, you can optimize many aspects of your "reproductive home" with DIY approaches.

This section explores practical, evidence-based strategies you can implement right away to enhance your fertility. These DIY improvements strengthen your reproductive foundation, upgrade your body's building materials, clean up your internal environment, and provide targeted support for your hormonal systems.

STRENGTHENING THE FRAME: STRESS REDUCTION TECHNIQUES

Stress is perhaps the most underappreciated factor affecting fertility. **I have said for years that stress is your body's biggest hormone hijacker.** Like a wooden frame that warps under pressure, your

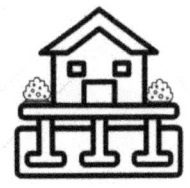

reproductive system can become distorted when chronic stress floods your body with cortisol and other stress hormones.

The Stress-Fertility Connection

Chronic stress impacts fertility through multiple mechanisms:
- **Hormonal Disruption:** Elevated cortisol can suppress reproductive hormone production, interfere with ovulation, and reduce testosterone in men
- **Blood Flow Reduction:** Stress triggers vasoconstriction, reducing blood flow to reproductive organs
- **Immune Dysregulation:** Stress alters immune function, potentially affecting implantation
- **Sleep Disruption:** Stress-related sleep problems further disrupt hormonal balance
- **Behavioral Changes:** Stress often leads to poor food choices, increased alcohol consumption, and reduced physical activity

Structural Reinforcement Techniques

These evidence-based approaches help reinforce your body's stress response system:

1. **Mind-Body Practices**
   - **Meditation:** Research shows that women practicing meditation show improved hormone levels and higher pregnancy rates during fertility treatments. Start with just 5–10 minutes daily using apps like Calm, Headspace, or Insight Timer.
   - **Progressive Muscle Relaxation:** This technique involves tensing and then releasing each muscle group, signaling to your nervous system that it's safe to relax.

Practice for 10–15 minutes before bed to improve sleep quality.
- **Guided Visualization:** Fertility-focused visualizations can reduce stress hormones and activate the parasympathetic nervous system. Try visualizing your reproductive organs functioning optimally, blood flowing freely to your uterus and ovaries, or your hormones in perfect balance.
- **Mindfulness-Based Stress Reduction (MBSR):** This structured eight-week program has been shown to normalize stress hormones and improve fertility outcomes. Look for local programs or online options.

2. Physical Stress Reduction
- **Fertility Yoga:** Specific yoga sequences can improve blood flow to reproductive organs, reduce stress hormones, and support hormonal balance. Focus on restorative poses like legs up the wall, supported bridge pose, and reclined bound angle pose.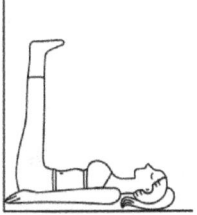
- **Acupressure Points:** Stimulating specific acupressure points can activate the parasympathetic nervous system and improve reproductive function. The points Liver 3 (between your big toe and second toe), Spleen 6 (four fingers above your inner ankle), and Conception Vessel 4 (three finger-widths below your navel) are particularly beneficial.

- **Heart Rate Variability Training:** Using devices like HeartMath or apps like Inner Balance, you can train your nervous system to maintain coherence between your heart and brain, reducing stress hormones and improving hormonal balance.
- **Nature Exposure:** Research shows that spending just 20–30 minutes in nature significantly reduces cortisol levels. Make daily outdoor time a priority, even if it's just sitting in your backyard or a local park. Get that Vitamin N (nature) in daily!

3. Stress-Proofing Your Schedule
- **Fertility-Friendly Time Management:** Prioritize activities that support your fertility and eliminate or delegate those that drain your energy.
- **Digital Detox Periods:** Set boundaries around technology use, especially in the evening, to reduce stress and improve sleep quality.
- **Pleasurable Activity Scheduling:** Intentionally schedule activities that bring you joy and relaxation—your reproductive system functions best when you feel safe and content.
- **"No" Practice:** Learning to decline commitments that increase your stress load is a crucial fertility skill. Practice saying no to at least one request each week.

> **Success Story:** Melissa, a 36-year-old marketing executive, had been trying to conceive for 18 months while working 60+ hour weeks. Her hormone testing showed elevated cortisol and irregular ovulation. After implementing a comprehensive stress reduction protocol—including morning meditation, twice-weekly restorative yoga, setting firm work boundaries, and regular nature walks—her cortisol normalized within three months, her cycles became regular, and she conceived naturally four months later.

ADVANCED NERVOUS SYSTEM REGULATION: THE SAFETY TO CONCEIVE

The Nervous System's Role in Fertility: Polyvagal Theory and the Safety to Conceive

In our home renovation metaphor, your nervous system functions as the master control panel that determines whether your home is in "security mode" or "welcome guests mode." Dr. Stephen Porges' Polyvagal Theory reveals that our reproductive system is intimately connected to our sense of safety and social connection. When we don't feel safe—whether physically, emotionally, or relationally—our

Structural Foundation Work

nervous system literally shuts down non-essential functions, including reproduction.

This isn't just psychological—it's deeply physiological. Your nervous system must signal "safety" before your body will invest energy in creating new life.

UNDERSTANDING THE THREE NEURAL PATHWAYS

Polyvagal Theory describes three distinct neural pathways that affect our state of being and, consequently, our fertility:

1. **The Social Engagement System (Ventral Vagal)**
    - **The "Safe and Connected" State:** This is the state where optimal fertility occurs
    - **Nervous System State:** Calm, connected, socially engaged
    - **Physical Markers:** Relaxed facial muscles, smooth breathing, regular heart rate variability
    - **Fertility Impact:** Optimal hormone production, healthy ovulation, receptive uterine environment
    - **Behavioral Signs:** Eye contact, prosodic voice, desire for intimacy and connection

2. **The Sympathetic System (Fight or Flight)**
    The "Mobilized for Danger" State: Chronic activation devastates fertility
    - **Nervous System State:** Alert, anxious, activated
    - **Physical Markers:** Rapid heart rate, shallow breathing, muscle tension
    - **Fertility Impact:** Elevated cortisol suppresses reproductive hormones, disrupts ovulation, reduces implantation success

- **Behavioral Signs:** Hypervigilance, difficulty relaxing, racing thoughts

3. **The Dorsal Vagal System (Freeze/Shutdown)**
   The "Immobilized by Fear" State: Represents the body's ultimate conservation mode
   - **Nervous System State:** Shut down, disconnected, hopeless
   - **Physical Markers:** Slowed heart rate, shallow breathing, digestive shutdown
   - **Fertility Impact:** Complete suppression of reproductive function, amenorrhea, loss of libido
   - **Behavioral Signs:** Depression, isolation, feeling "stuck" or hopeless

THE FERTILITY SAFETY ASSESSMENT

Your body continuously performs an unconscious "safety assessment" through a process called **neuroception**—the subconscious detection of safety or threat. This assessment happens below conscious awareness but profoundly impacts reproductive function.

FACTORS THAT SIGNAL "UNSAFE" TO YOUR NERVOUS SYSTEM:

- Chronic relationship conflict or emotional disconnection from partner
- Financial insecurity or work-related stress
- Unresolved trauma (including medical trauma from fertility treatments and birth trauma)
- Perfectionism and chronic self-criticism
- Social isolation or lack of supportive community
- Environmental chaos or unpredictability

- History of loss (pregnancy loss, death of loved ones, major life changes)
- Chronic illness or pain
- Toxic relationships or abusive dynamics

THE BODY'S MEMORY OF BIRTH TRAUMA

My own experience illustrates how powerfully birth trauma can signal "unsafe" to our nervous systems, affecting not just our willingness but our body's readiness to conceive again. My first birth was profoundly traumatic—after a long labor, I developed chorioamnionitis and required an emergency C-section, followed by a devastating two-liter postpartum hemorrhage. For anyone who has experienced postpartum hemorrhage, you know the terror that accompanies watching your life force literally drain away. My husband witnessed this blood loss while holding our newborn son in recovery, so the situation traumatized both of us. I required blood transfusions and was so weakened by the experience that initially, neither of us wanted to attempt pregnancy again. Yet, as many mothers know all too well, regardless of how traumatic delivery was, once you hold that beautiful baby, we somehow think we forget what we went through and find ourselves wanting to do it again. While my mind was ready to try for a second child relatively quickly, I now wonder if my body wasn't.

Looking back, I suspect part of my fertility struggles was that I hadn't worked through the trauma of my first birth—my nervous system was still signaling "unsafe" for pregnancy and delivery. The year I finally conceived Michael, I intentionally took time to process that birth trauma, preparing both my mind and body for what could potentially happen again. Even though doctors reassured me that repeat hemorrhage was very unlikely, and I had placenta previa requiring a scheduled 36-week C-section (eliminating labor and its associated hemorrhage risks), I knew I needed to do the internal work regardless. Mentally, I felt prepared and safe going into my second delivery. Unfortunately, I lost three liters that time, and it was even more challenging—but that's another story. The point is that our bodies hold the memory of trauma, and until we address it, our nervous systems may continue sending "unsafe" signals that can impact both fertility and birth outcomes.

Factors That Signal "SAFE" to Your Nervous System:
- Secure, supportive, intimate relationship
- Consistent daily routines and predictability
- Strong social support network
- Financial stability and security
- Safe, calm physical environment
- Regular co-regulation with trusted others
- Playfulness and joy in daily life
- Connection to nature and grounding practices
- Meaning and purpose beyond fertility
- Regulated nervous system in your partner

THE CO-REGULATION CONNECTION

One of the most powerful aspects of Polyvagal Theory for fertility is understanding **co-regulation**—how we use connection with others to regulate our nervous systems. Your partner's nervous system state directly influences yours, and vice versa.

Creating Co-Regulation for Fertility:
- **Synchronized breathing** exercises with your partner
- **Eye contact and gentle touch** without sexual agenda

- **Shared calming activities** like walking, cooking, or listening to music together
- **Vocal toning or humming** together (stimulates vagal tone)
- **Playful interactions** that create joy and safety
- **Regular check-ins** about emotional states without trying to "fix" each other

VAGAL NERVE STIMULATION: ACTIVATING YOUR SAFETY SYSTEM

The vagus nerve is the primary pathway of the parasympathetic nervous system and can be specifically stimulated to enhance the "safety" signal to your reproductive system.

NATURAL VAGAL NERVE STIMULATION TECHNIQUES

Breathing-Based Stimulation:
- **Extended Exhale Breathing:** Inhale for 4 counts, exhale for 8 counts
- **Coherent Breathing:** 5 seconds in, 5 seconds out for 5–10 minutes
- **Bee Breath (Bhramari):** Humming while breathing to create vagal vibration
- **Cold Water Face Immersion:** Activates the dive reflex and vagal stimulation

Vocal Stimulation:
- **Singing or Humming:** Creates vibrations that stimulate the vagus nerve
- **Gargling:** Simple daily practice that activates vagal pathways
- **Chanting or Vocal Toning:** Especially effective when done with partner
- **Laughter:** Authentic laughter naturally stimulates vagal tone

Physical Stimulation:
- **Gentle Neck Massage:** Focus on the sides of the neck where the vagus nerve runs
- **Ear Massage:** The vagus nerve has branches in the ear
- **Yoga Poses:** Child's pose, legs up the wall, supported fish pose
- **Progressive Muscle Relaxation:** Systematic tension and release

TECHNOLOGY-ASSISTED VAGAL STIMULATION

Vagal Nerve Stimulator Devices: Modern technology offers several options for targeted vagal stimulation:

Consumer-Grade Devices:
- **Apollo Neuro:** Wearable device that delivers gentle vibrations to improve heart rate variability
- **Sensate:** Infrasonic resonance device placed on chest to stimulate vagal pathways
- **HeartMath Inner Balance:** Biofeedback device that trains heart rate variability
- **Muse Headband:** Meditation device that provides real-time brainwave feedback
- **Pulsetto:** Neck-worn vagal nerve stimulation device that uses electrical pulses to activate the vagus nerve, specifically designed for stress reduction and nervous system regulation

I actually started with the Apollo Neuro but switched to the Pulsetto, and I hum or sing on the way to work!

Clinical Devices (require practitioner):
- **Auricular Vagal Nerve Stimulation:** Ear-based electrical stimulation
- **Transcutaneous Vagal Nerve Stimulation (tVNS):** Non-invasive electrical stimulation

IMPORTANT CONSIDERATIONS:
- Start with natural techniques before investing in devices
- Consistency matters more than intensity
- Work with practitioners experienced in both fertility and nervous system regulation
- Not all devices are appropriate during pregnancy

CREATING YOUR PERSONAL SAFETY PROTOCOL
Daily Safety-Building Practices:

Morning Safety Activation:
- Five minutes of coherent breathing upon waking
- Gratitude practice focusing on relationships and security
- Gentle movement or stretching
- Positive affirmations about your body's wisdom

Throughout the Day:
- Regular check-ins with your nervous system state
- Micro-moments of co-regulation with partner or trusted friends
- Nature connection, even if just viewing trees from a window
- Humming or singing while doing routine tasks

Evening Safety Consolidation:
- Partner connection time without discussing fertility stress
- Warm bath or shower (activates parasympathetic response)
- Gentle self-massage or partner massage
- Technology-assisted vagal stimulation, if using devices

Weekly Safety Reinforcement:
- Dedicated time in nature
- Social connection with supportive friends or family
- Creative or playful activities
- Professional support (therapy, massage, acupuncture)

THE FERTILITY-SAFETY TIMELINE

Understanding the nervous system's role in fertility helps explain why:
- Some women conceive immediately after reducing work stress or relationship conflict
- Fertility often improves during vacations or periods of reduced responsibility
- Many couples conceive after "giving up" trying (nervous system finally feels safe to let go of control)
- Trauma-informed therapy can dramatically improve fertility outcomes
- Social support groups often correlate with higher pregnancy rates

PARTNER NERVOUS SYSTEM CONSIDERATIONS

Male nervous system states also significantly impact fertility:
- Chronic stress reduces testosterone and sperm quality
- Nervous system dysregulation affects libido and sexual function

- Partner's anxiety can dysregulate female partner's nervous system
- Co-regulation practices benefit both partners' reproductive health

Creating Couple Nervous System Safety:
- Practice breathing exercises together
- Create predictable rhythms and routines
- Address relationship conflicts with professional support if needed
- Engage in non-fertility-focused intimacy regularly
- Share household and emotional burdens equitably

WHEN PROFESSIONAL SUPPORT IS NEEDED

Consider nervous system-focused therapy when:
- Fertility treatments are creating more trauma than support
- Relationship stress is chronic despite good intentions
- History of trauma (sexual, medical, emotional) affecting intimacy
- Chronic anxiety or depression impacting daily function
- Feeling disconnected from your body or partner
- Obsessive thoughts about fertility consuming daily life

Types of Nervous System-Informed Therapy:
- Somatic Experiencing for trauma resolution
- EMDR for processing fertility-related trauma
- Polyvagal-informed therapy for nervous system regulation
- Gottman Method couples therapy for relationship safety
- Internal Family Systems for addressing internal conflict

THE ULTIMATE FERTILITY TRUTH

Your nervous system needs to believe it's safe to bring a child into your current life situation. This isn't about having perfect circumstances—it's about your internal sense of safety, connection, and capacity to welcome new life.

Sometimes the most powerful fertility intervention isn't another supplement or treatment—it's creating genuine safety and connection in your daily life. When your nervous system finally signals "safe," your reproductive system often responds with surprising speed and effectiveness.

In our home renovation metaphor, this means ensuring your home's security system is signaling "welcome" rather than "threat detected" before expecting your reproductive systems to function optimally. The most beautifully renovated home won't welcome guests if the alarm system is constantly activated.

CHAPTER 18

QUALITY MATERIALS—NUTRITION AND EGG QUALITY ENHANCEMENT

QUALITY MATERIALS: NUTRITIONAL OPTIMIZATION FOR FERTILITY

Just as a home renovation requires quality building materials, your body needs optimal nutritional components to build healthy eggs, sperm, hormones, and eventually, a baby. Nutrition forms the literal building blocks of your fertility.

Before we dive into food recommendations, I have to pause to share the dangers of seed oils here...

SEED OILS: THE HIDDEN EGG AND SPERM QUALITY DESTROYERS

In our home renovation metaphor, industrial seed oils are like using cheap, toxic building materials that compromise the structural integrity of your entire project. While they may seem cost-effective and convenient, these highly processed oils create widespread oxidative damage that specifically targets the delicate cellular components essential for reproduction—particularly the mitochondria in eggs and sperm.

THE OXIDATIVE DAMAGE CONNECTION

Eggs and sperm are among the most metabolically active cells in the human body, requiring enormous amounts of cellular energy to function properly. This energy production occurs in the mitochondria—the cellular powerhouses—which are extremely vulnerable to oxidative damage from industrial seed oils.

HOW SEED OILS DAMAGE REPRODUCTIVE CELLS:

- **Lipid Peroxidation:** Seed oils are rich in omega-6 fatty acids that become rancid when heated, creating toxic aldehydes that damage cellular membranes
- **Mitochondrial Dysfunction:** These toxic compounds specifically target mitochondria, reducing energy production in eggs and sperm
- **DNA Fragmentation:** Oxidative stress from seed oils increases DNA damage in both eggs and sperm, leading to poor embryo quality and increased miscarriage risk
- **Inflammatory Cascade:** Excess omega-6 fatty acids trigger systemic inflammation that disrupts hormonal signaling and implantation
- **Membrane Instability:** Poor-quality fats get incorporated into cell membranes, making them less flexible and functional

The most concerning aspect is that once these damaged fats are incorporated into your cell membranes, it can take months to replace them with healthier alternatives—which aligns perfectly with the three- or four-month timeline for egg and sperm development.

INDUSTRIAL SEED OILS TO ELIMINATE

These oils are highly processed, often rancid, and inflammatory. Avoid them completely during your fertility journey:

Primary Offenders:
- **Soybean oil** (most common in processed foods)
- **Canola oil** (rapeseed oil)
- **Corn oil**
- **Sunflower oil**
- **Safflower oil**
- **Cottonseed oil**
- **Grapeseed oil**
- **Rice bran oil**

Hidden Sources to Watch For:
- Most salad dressings and mayonnaise
- Fried foods at restaurants
- Packaged snacks and crackers
- Conventional nuts and seeds (often roasted in seed oils)
- Protein bars and processed health foods
- Most conventional cooking sprays
- Many "healthy" products marketed as plant-based alternatives

Restaurant and Food Service Reality: The vast majority of restaurants use soybean or canola oil for cooking, making dining out a significant source of seed oil exposure. Even "healthy" restaurants often use these oils unless they specifically advertise otherwise.

FERTILITY-SUPPORTING FAT ALTERNATIVES

These traditional fats have nourished human reproduction for thousands of years and support optimal cellular function:

Animal-Based Fats (excellent for high-heat cooking):
- **Grass-fed beef tallow:** Rich in fat-soluble vitamins and extremely stable at high temperatures
- **Grass-fed butter and ghee:** Contains vitamin K2, CLA, and other fertility-supporting compounds
- **Pastured lard:** High in vitamin D and stable saturated fats
- **Duck fat:** Excellent for roasting vegetables and adds rich flavor

Plant-Based Alternatives:
- **Extra virgin olive oil:** Use for low-heat cooking and dressings (avoid heating to smoking point)
- **Avocado oil:** High smoke point, suitable for higher-heat cooking
- **Coconut oil:** Contains lauric acid and other antimicrobial compounds
- **MCT oil:** Provides quick energy and supports brain function

Specialty Options:
- **Macadamia nut oil:** Low in omega-6, suitable for cooking
- **Red palm oil:** Rich in vitamin E and carotenoids (ensure sustainably sourced)

THE OMEGA-6 TO OMEGA-3 RATIO PROBLEM

Our ancestors consumed omega-6 to omega-3 fatty acids in a ratio of approximately 1:1 to 4:1. The modern Western diet, heavily laden with seed oils, creates ratios of 20:1 or even higher, leading to:

- Chronic systemic inflammation
- Impaired hormone production
- Reduced egg and sperm quality
- Compromised implantation environment
- Increased risk of pregnancy complications

PRACTICAL IMPLEMENTATION STRATEGY

Phase 1: Elimination (Weeks 1–4)

- Clean out your pantry of all products containing seed oils
- Learn to read ingredient labels carefully
- Begin cooking primarily at home, using approved fats
- Find seed oil-free alternatives for frequently used products

Phase 2: Replacement (Weeks 5–8)

- Stock kitchen with high-quality cooking fats
- Identify restaurants that use healthier cooking oils
- Experiment with new cooking techniques using traditional fats
- Make homemade versions of commonly used condiments

Phase 3: Optimization (Weeks 9–12)

- Focus on balancing omega-6 to omega-3 ratios
- Increase omega-3-rich foods (wild-caught fish, grass-fed meat, walnuts)
- Consider high-quality fish oil supplementation

- Monitor improvements in energy, skin quality, and overall inflammation

RESEARCH SUPPORT

Studies consistently show that dietary fat quality directly impacts reproductive outcomes:

- Research published in *Human Reproduction* found that women consuming the highest amounts of omega-6 fatty acids had significantly lower IVF success rates.[3]
- A study in *Fertility and Sterility* demonstrated that men with higher omega-3 to omega-6 ratios had better sperm morphology and concentration.[4]
- Multiple studies link seed oil consumption to increased inflammation markers that negatively impact fertility.

HOME COOKING TRANSFORMATION

Making this shift requires embracing home cooking, but the fertility benefits are profound:

- **High-Heat Cooking:** Use tallow, ghee, or coconut oil for sautéing, roasting, and frying
- **Medium-Heat Cooking:** Avocado oil works well for most stovetop cooking
- **Low-Heat and Raw Applications:** Extra virgin olive oil for dressings and finishing dishes
- **Baking:** Coconut oil, butter, or ghee, depending on desired flavor profile

---

[3] Chiu, Y.H., Karmon, A.E., Gaskins, A.J., Arvizu, M., Williams, P.L., Souter, I., Rueda, B.R., Hauser, R., Chavarro, J.E. (2018). Serum omega-3 fatty acids and treatment outcomes among women undergoing assisted reproduction. *Human Reproduction*, 33(1), 156-165.

[4] Safarinejad, M.R. (2011). Relationship of omega-3 and omega-6 fatty acids with semen characteristics, and anti-oxidant status of seminal plasma: A comparison between fertile and infertile men. *Clinical Nutrition*, 30(6), 796-804.

THE TIMELINE CONNECTION

I'll be honest, reducing seed oils has been one of the hardest challenges for me, but remember that the fats you consume today become part of your cellular membranes within weeks; however, it takes 3–4 months to fully replace the fatty acid composition of your cells. This timeline perfectly aligns with egg and sperm development, making fat-quality optimization one of the most impactful changes you can make for fertility.

Just as you wouldn't use water-damaged wood or toxic materials in a home renovation, eliminating inflammatory seed oils while embracing traditional, nourishing fats provides the high-quality building blocks your reproductive cells need to function optimally. This single dietary change can significantly reduce oxidative stress, improve cellular energy production, and create a more favorable environment for conception and healthy pregnancy.

FERTILITY FOUNDATION NUTRITION

Okay, now for more general recommendations, the core nutritional approach for fertility focuses on:

- **A High-Quality Prenatal Vitamin:** Start with a comprehensive, methylated prenatal containing folate (not folic acid), adequate B vitamins, and bioavailable minerals as your nutritional foundation—even before you're actively trying to conceive
- **Anti-Inflammatory Foods:** Chronic inflammation can disrupt hormone balance and egg/sperm quality. Emphasize fatty fish, olive oil, colorful fruits and vegetables, nuts, seeds, and spices like turmeric and ginger.
- **Blood Sugar Stability:** Insulin resistance and blood sugar fluctuations disrupt ovulation and hormone production.

Include protein and healthy fat with every meal, minimize refined carbohydrates, and space meals 4–5 hours apart.

- **Hormone-Supporting Fats:** Cholesterol and essential fatty acids are required for hormone production. Include sources of omega-3 fatty acids (wild-caught fish, walnuts, flaxseeds), as well as saturated fats from quality sources (grass-fed butter, coconut oil).
- **Micronutrient Density:** Focus on nutrient-rich foods to provide the vitamins and minerals essential for reproductive function—dark leafy greens, organ meats, egg yolks, sea vegetables, and colorful vegetables and fruits.
- **Detoxification Support:** Include foods that support liver function and detoxification, such as cruciferous vegetables (broccoli, cauliflower, Brussels sprouts), artichokes, beets, and fresh herbs.
- **Individualization:** Adjust your nutrition based on personal food sensitivities, health conditions, and metabolic needs. Many people benefit from eliminating gluten and dairy temporarily to reduce inflammation.

EGG QUALITY ENHANCEMENT: OPTIMIZING YOUR MOST PRECIOUS RESOURCE

In our home renovation metaphor, egg quality represents the foundation materials for your most important construction project—creating new life. Just as you wouldn't build a house with substandard materials, optimizing egg quality ensures you're working with the best possible foundation for conception and healthy pregnancy.

Unlike men, who produce new sperm every 74 days, women are born with all the eggs they'll ever have. However, the quality of those eggs—their energy production, DNA integrity, and developmental potential—can be significantly influenced by the environment you create in your body during the crucial 100 days before ovulation.

UNDERSTANDING EGG QUALITY: BEYOND THE NUMBERS

When we talk about egg quality, we're referring to several critical factors:

Chromosomal Integrity:
- Proper chromosome number (46 total: 23 from egg, 23 from sperm)
- Intact DNA structure without fragmentation
- Ability to combine genetic material successfully with sperm

Mitochondrial Function:
- Adequate energy production for fertilization and early embryo development
- Healthy mitochondrial DNA
- Sufficient mitochondrial numbers to support cellular processes

Cytoplasmic Maturity:
- Proper protein content to support early embryo development
- Appropriate enzyme levels for cellular division
- Optimal cellular organization and structure

Developmental Potential:
- Ability to fertilize successfully
- Capacity to develop into a healthy blastocyst
- Potential to implant and grow into a healthy baby

THE 100-DAY OPPORTUNITY WINDOW

Here's the encouraging truth: while you can't create new eggs, you have a powerful 100-day window to influence the quality of eggs approaching ovulation. During this time, eggs undergo their final maturation process, and the environment you create in your body directly impacts their development.

THE EGG DEVELOPMENT TIMELINE:
- **Day 1–70:** Early follicular development begins
- **Day 70–85:** Rapid growth and maturation phase
- **Day 85–100:** Final maturation and preparation for ovulation
- **Day 100:** Ovulation and potential fertilization

This means the egg you ovulate this month began its final development journey over three months ago, and the egg you'll ovulate three months from now is beginning that journey today. Your nutrition, stress levels, sleep quality, and overall health during these 100 days will directly influence egg quality.

COMPREHENSIVE EGG QUALITY ENHANCEMENT PROTOCOL
PHASE 1: MITOCHONDRIAL POWERHOUSE SUPPORT (MONTHS 1–3)

CoQ10 (as Ubiquinol): 600–800mg daily
- The most researched supplement for egg quality
- Provides energy for cellular processes and acts as powerful antioxidant
- Take with fat-containing meals in divided doses
- Choose Ubiquinol form for better absorption

PQQ (Pyrroloquinoline Quinone): 10–20mg daily
- Stimulates growth of new mitochondria
- Enhances existing mitochondrial function
- Take on empty stomach for best absorption

NAC (N-Acetyl Cysteine): 600mg twice daily
- Powerful antioxidant that supports glutathione production
- Shown to improve egg quality markers in research
- Take on empty stomach

Alpha-Lipoic Acid: 300mg twice daily
- Regenerates other antioxidants
- Supports mitochondrial function and glucose metabolism
- Take with meals

PHASE 2: ADVANCED ANTIOXIDANT PROTECTION (MONTH 2-3)

Vitamin E (Mixed Tocopherols): 400 IU daily
- Protects cell membranes from oxidative damage
- Avoid synthetic forms (dl-alpha tocopherol)
- Take with fat-containing meal

Vitamin C: 1,000mg twice daily
- Water-soluble antioxidant that works synergistically with vitamin E
- Supports collagen formation and immune function
- Take with meals to reduce GI upset

Resveratrol: 100–200mg daily
- Activates sirtuins (longevity proteins)
- May improve egg quality through cellular protection
- Take on empty stomach for best absorption

Astaxanthin: 12mg daily
- One of the most powerful antioxidants
- Crosses cellular membranes to protect mitochondria
- Take with fat for absorption

PHASE 3: HORMONAL AND METABOLIC SUPPORT (THROUGHOUT)

Vitamin D3: 4,000–5,000 IU daily
- Critical for hormone production and immune function
- Many women are severely deficient
- Target blood levels: 50–80 ng/mL

Omega-3 Fatty Acids: 2–3g daily (EPA/DHA)
- Essential for cell membrane integrity
- Anti-inflammatory effects
- Choose molecularly distilled, third-party tested

Melatonin: 3mg before bed
- Powerful antioxidant that concentrates in follicular fluid
- Supports sleep quality (critical for hormone production)
- May directly protect eggs from oxidative damage

Folate (as Methylfolate): 800mcg daily
- Essential for DNA synthesis and repair
- Choose active form, especially if MTHFR variants
- Critical during conception and early pregnancy

ADVANCED STRATEGIES FOR ENHANCED RESULTS
DIETARY OPTIMIZATION FOR EGG QUALITY

The Mediterranean Fertility Diet: Research consistently shows that women following Mediterranean dietary patterns have better egg quality markers and higher IVF success rates.

Key Components:
- **High-quality protein:** Wild-caught fish, grass-fed meats, pasture-raised eggs
- **Healthy fats:** Extra virgin olive oil, avocados, nuts, seeds
- **Antioxidant-rich vegetables:** Colorful produce, especially dark leafy greens
- **Complex carbohydrates:** Quinoa, sweet potatoes, ancient grains
- **Anti-inflammatory spices:** Turmeric, ginger, garlic, herbs

Foods to Eliminate:
- **Processed foods and refined sugars** (increase inflammation and oxidative stress)
- **Trans fats and industrial seed oils** (damage cell membranes)
- **Excessive caffeine** (more than 200mg daily may affect egg quality)
- **Alcohol** (toxic to developing eggs)
- **High-mercury fish** (tuna, swordfish, king mackerel)

LIFESTYLE FACTORS THAT IMPACT EGG QUALITY
Sleep Optimization:
- **7–9 hours nightly** for optimal hormone production
- **Consistent sleep schedule** to support circadian rhythm

- **Dark, cool sleeping environment** to maximize melatonin production
- **No screens 1–2 hours before bed** to prevent melatonin suppression

Exercise Balance:
- **Moderate exercise enhances egg quality** through improved circulation and hormone balance
- **Excessive high-intensity exercise can be detrimental** by increasing oxidative stress
- **Optimal approach:** 30–45 minutes of moderate activity 5–6 days weekly
- **Include strength training** to support hormone production and metabolism

Stress Management:
- **Chronic stress elevates cortisol,** which can interfere with reproductive hormones
- **Daily stress reduction practices:** meditation, yoga, deep breathing
- **Heart rate variability training** to improve stress resilience
- **Regular nature exposure** to reduce cortisol and support overall well-being

ENVIRONMENTAL OPTIMIZATION

Reduce Exposure to Endocrine Disruptors:
- **Plastics:** Use glass or stainless steel for food storage and water bottles

- **Personal care products:** Choose clean, non-toxic alternatives
- **Household cleaners:** Switch to natural or DIY options
- **Air quality:** Use HEPA air purifiers, especially in bedroom
- **Water quality:** Install high-quality filtration systems

EMF Reduction:
- **Limit cell phone exposure** near reproductive organs
- **Turn off Wi-Fi at night** or use timer switches
- **Avoid laptop directly on lap** when working
- **Create EMF-free sleeping environment** when possible

ADVANCED ANTIOXIDANT SUPPORT: EMERGING OPTIONS
C60 (Carbon 60): The Molecular Antioxidant

C60 represents a cutting-edge approach to antioxidant support with unique properties that may benefit egg quality:

What Makes C60 Special:
- **Molecular cage structure** allows it to neutralize multiple free radicals continuously
- **Cellular penetration** may reach areas other antioxidants cannot access
- **Mitochondrial protection** particularly relevant for energy-demanding eggs
- **Sustained activity** unlike traditional antioxidants that become depleted

My Personal Experience: Between my first and second IVF cycles, I incorporated C60 into my comprehensive antioxidant protocol.

The results were dramatic—my euploid embryo rate improved from 33% to 56%, far above the expected average for my age. While I cannot attribute this solely to C60, the timing and magnitude of improvement suggest my intensive antioxidant approach, which included C60, played a significant role.

Considerations for C60:
- **Quality matters:** Choose reputable manufacturers with third-party testing
- **Timing:** Begin 3–4 months before conception attempts
- **Integration:** Use as part of comprehensive protocol, not standalone
- **Professional guidance:** Discuss with healthcare provider familiar with emerging supplements

Age-Specific Strategies
Women Under 35:
- **Focus on prevention** of oxidative damage
- **Basic antioxidant protocol** often sufficient
- **Emphasize lifestyle optimization** and environmental cleanup
- **3-month preparation timeline** typically adequate

Women 35–40:
- **More intensive antioxidant support** recommended
- **Consider advanced supplements** like CoQ10 at higher doses
- **Six-month preparation timeline** may be beneficial
- **Regular monitoring** of progress through cycle tracking

Women Over 40:
- **Maximum antioxidant support** often warranted
- **Consider all advanced strategies,** including emerging options
- **Longer preparation timeline** (6+ months) may be needed
- **Integration with medical treatment** often beneficial
- **For women with POF or very low ovarian reserve,** see specialized protocols in chapter 12

INTEGRATION WITH FERTILITY TREATMENTS
Preparing for IVF
3–4 Months Before Cycle:
- Begin comprehensive egg quality protocol
- Optimize all lifestyle factors
- Complete environmental detoxification
- Establish stress management practices

During IVF Stimulation:
- Continue antioxidant support (coordinate with Reproductive Endocrinologist)
- Some supplements may need modification during medications
- Maintain sleep and stress management practices
- Focus on anti-inflammatory nutrition

Post-Retrieval:
- Support recovery with continued antioxidants
- Prepare for transfer with implantation-supporting nutrients
- Maintain all lifestyle optimizations

Natural Conception Enhancement
- **Full 100-day optimization** before active conception attempts
- **Continue protocol** throughout conception attempts
- **Cycle-specific modifications** based on fertility awareness methods
- **Monitor improvements** through cycle quality and energy levels

MEASURING PROGRESS

Subjective Improvements (Often noticed within 4–8 weeks):
- **Increased energy levels** throughout cycle
- **Improved sleep quality** and mood stability
- **Better cycle regularity** and reduced PMS symptoms
- **Enhanced exercise recovery** and overall vitality

Objective Measurements (3–6 months):
- **AMH levels** (may improve modestly with optimization)
- **Cycle length and regularity** improvements
- **Ovulation quality** (confirmed through BBT, progesterone testing)
- **IVF outcomes** (if applicable): egg quality, fertilization rates, embryo development

When to Reassess Protocol:
- **No subjective improvements after 8 weeks** of full protocol
- **Worsening cycle quality** despite optimization efforts
- **New symptoms** or intolerance to supplements
- **Achieving pregnancy** (transition to pregnancy-specific protocols)

THE TIMELINE REALITY

Remember that egg quality optimization requires patience and consistency. The eggs you're working to improve today won't be ovulated for 3-4 months. This biological reality means:

- **Immediate changes** in supplements and lifestyle begin protecting future eggs
- **Full benefits** typically seen after 3–6 months of consistent optimization
- **Continued improvements** may occur with longer protocols
- **Pregnancy preparation** ideally begins 6+ months before conception attempts

SUCCESS STORIES AND HOPE

The research on egg quality improvement is encouraging. Studies show that comprehensive antioxidant protocols can:

- **Improve fertilization rates** in IVF by 20–30%
- **Increase blastocyst formation** and embryo quality
- **Enhance natural conception rates** in women over 35
- **Reduce miscarriage rates** by supporting chromosomal integrity

My own experience demonstrates the potential for dramatic improvement. The difference between my IVF cycles—from 33% to 56% euploid embryos—shows that even in cases where conventional medicine suggests limited options, comprehensive optimization can create remarkable results.

Your eggs have been with you since before birth, but their quality isn't fixed. In the 100 days before ovulation, you have a powerful opportunity to provide them with the best possible environment for optimal development. This window of opportunity exists every cycle, offering hope and the possibility for improvement regardless of age or previous challenges.

By implementing these egg quality enhancement strategies, you're not just improving your chances of conception—you're potentially influencing the health of your future child from the very moment of fertilization. The investment you make in egg quality today may be one of the most important gifts you can give to your growing family.

FOUNDATION REINFORCEMENT: IV THERAPY OPTIONS

For some individuals, oral supplementation isn't sufficient to overcome significant nutrient deficiencies or increased demands. IV therapy delivers nutrients directly to the bloodstream, bypassing digestive limitations:

- **Nutrient IV Therapy:** Customized IV formulations can rapidly replenish key fertility nutrients like vitamin C, B vitamins, magnesium, zinc, and glutathione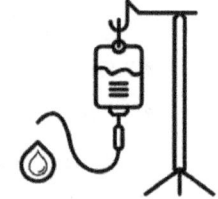
- **When to Consider IV Support:**
    - If you have diagnosed absorption issues (celiac disease, inflammatory bowel disease, etc.)
    - When comprehensive testing shows significant nutrient deficiencies
    - During intensive detoxification protocols
    - For rapid nutritional support before fertility treatments
    - When preparing for embryo transfer or implantation

- **Common Fertility IV Formulations:**
    - Myers Cocktail with added fertility nutrients
    - Glutathione IVs for detoxification support

- Vitamin C IVs for immune modulation and egg quality
- NAD+ IVs for cellular energy and DNA repair

Clinical Pearl: IV therapy should complement, not replace, a nutrient-dense diet and oral supplementation. Work with a practitioner experienced in both fertility and IV therapy for proper customization.

STRUCTURAL INTEGRITY: GUT HEALTH FOR OVERALL SYSTEM SUPPORT

Your gut isn't just responsible for digesting food—it's integral to hormone metabolism, immune function, inflammation regulation, and nutrient absorption. A compromised gut can undermine even the best fertility protocol.

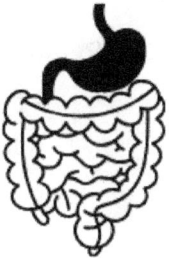

THE GUT-FERTILITY CONNECTION

- **Estrobolome:** The collection of gut bacteria that metabolize estrogens, influencing whether estrogens are recycled or eliminated
- **Intestinal Barrier:** Prevents inflammatory substances from entering circulation and triggering systemic inflammation
- **Nutrient Absorption:** Ensures vitamins, minerals, and other nutrients reach your reproductive organs
- **Immune Regulation:** Balances immune function to allow proper implantation and pregnancy maintenance

Gut Restoration Protocol (as discussed in great detail in chapter 1 of *Your Longevity Blueprint*)

1. **Remove:**
   - Inflammatory foods (through elimination diet if necessary)

- Infections (bacterial, fungal, parasitic)
- Irritants (alcohol, NSAIDs, excess sugar)

2. **Replace:**
   - Digestive enzymes, if needed
   - Stomach acid support (apple cider vinegar or betaine HCl if appropriate)
   - Bile support for fat digestion (dandelion, artichoke, milk thistle)

3. **Reinoculate:**
   - Probiotic-rich foods (sauerkraut, kimchi, kefir if tolerated)
   - Specific probiotic strains (L. rhamnosus, L. acidophilus, B. longum)
   - Prebiotic foods to feed beneficial bacteria (garlic, onions, asparagus, dandelion greens)

4. **Repair:**
   - L-glutamine for intestinal cell regeneration
   - Zinc to support tight junction integrity
   - Bone broth for amino acids and collagen
   - Aloe vera, marshmallow root, and slippery elm for mucosal healing

5. **Rebalance:**
   - Manage stress, sleep, and exercise

Success Story: James and Diana had been trying to conceive for three years with unexplained infertility. Comprehensive testing revealed intestinal permeability ("leaky gut") in both partners, with elevated inflammatory markers and signs of poor nutrient absorption. After a 90-day gut restoration protocol, including elimination of gluten, dairy, and sugar, targeted supplements, and probiotic therapy, their inflammatory markers normalized, nutrient levels improved, and Diana conceived in the next three months.

CHAPTER 19

COMPLETE ENVIRONMENTAL AND NUTRITIONAL OPTIMIZATION

ENVIRONMENTAL CLEANUP: DETOXIFICATION FOR REPRODUCTIVE HEALTH

Just as you wouldn't renovate a home without first removing mold, asbestos, or lead paint, optimizing your fertility requires addressing the accumulated environmental toxins that disrupt hormonal function. In today's world, everyone carries a "body burden" of chemicals that can interfere with conception and healthy pregnancy.

THE TOXIN-FERTILITY CONNECTION

Research shows clear links between environmental toxins and fertility:

- **Endocrine Disruptors:** Chemicals that mimic or block natural hormones, including BPA, phthalates, pesticides, and flame retardants

- **Heavy Metals:** Mercury, lead, cadmium, and aluminum that damage egg and sperm quality
- **Air Pollutants:** Particulate matter and VOCs that increase inflammation and oxidative stress
- **Electromagnetic Fields (EMF):** Non-ionizing radiation that may affect cellular function and hormone signaling
- **Mold and Mycotoxins:** aflatoxin, gliotoxin, ochratoxin, trichothecenes, zearalenone

PURIFYING THE AIR AND WATER: CLEAN HOME ENVIRONMENT

Your home environment significantly impacts your reproductive health:

- **Water Filtration:**
    - Install a high-quality water filter for drinking and cooking (reverse osmosis plus remineralization is ideal)
    - Consider a shower filter to reduce chlorine and other contaminants absorbed through skin and lungs
    - Replace plastic water bottles with glass or stainless steel

- **Air Purification:**
    - Use HEPA air purifiers in bedroom and main living areas that filter down to small enough size for mold/mycotoxins
        » I like the purifiers made by AirDoctor,® but there are many great brands available
    - Maintain indoor plants that naturally filter air (spider plants, peace lilies, snake plants)

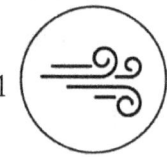

- o Open windows daily when possible for fresh air exchange
- o Remove shoes at the door to reduce indoor pollutants
- o Consider professional testing for mold if you suspect exposure

- **Home Detoxification:**
  - o Switch to natural cleaning products or make your own with vinegar, baking soda, and essential oils
  - o Replace chemical air fresheners with essential oil diffusers
  - o Choose furniture without flame retardants when possible
  - o Vacuum with a HEPA filter regularly to reduce dust (which harbors chemicals)
  - o Maintain humidity between 40-50% to discourage mold growth

NON-TOXIC BUILDING MATERIALS: SAFE PERSONAL CARE PRODUCTS

What you put on your body is as important as what you put in it:

- **Fertility-Friendly Personal Care:**
  - o Replace conventional products with clean alternatives (EWG's Skin Deep® database can help)
  - o Prioritize replacing products that remain on the skin (moisturizers, sunscreen) or cover large areas
  - o Pay special attention to intimacy products (lubricants, feminine hygiene)
    - » Use olive or coconut oil instead

- Look beyond "natural" marketing claims to actual ingredients

- **Key Ingredients to Avoid:**
    - Parabens (methylparaben, propylparaben)
    - Phthalates (often hidden in "fragrance")
    - Triclosan (antibacterial agent)
    - Chemical sunscreens (oxybenzone, avobenzone)
    - Sodium lauryl sulfate (foaming agent)
    - Synthetic fragrances

- **Menstrual Product Considerations:**
    - Switch to organic cotton tampons and pads or menstrual cups
    - Avoid scented products and plastic applicators
    - Consider period underwear made with OEKO-TEX certified fabrics
        » These are textiles that have been tested and certified to be free from harmful substances

SITE REMEDIATION: HEAVY METAL AND EMF REDUCTION

More intensive detoxification strategies can help reduce your body's toxic burden:

- **Heavy Metal Detoxification:**
    - Testing: Hair analysis, urine challenge tests, or blood tests to assess levels
    - Support binding and elimination with chlorella, cilantro, modified citrus pectin

- Ensure adequate sulfur compounds (NAC, MSM, glutathione)
- Use infrared sauna sessions to enhance excretion through sweat
- Always support detoxification with adequate hydration and electrolytes
- Pharmaceutical chelation is sometimes needed

- **EMF Reduction Strategies:**
  - Keep phones away from reproductive organs (not in pockets near testes or ovaries)
  - Turn devices to airplane mode when not in use, especially while sleeping
  - Unplug Wi-Fi router at night or use timer switch
  - Use wired connections instead of wireless when possible
  - Consider EMF shielding for bedroom if testing shows high levels

Important Note: Intensive detoxification should be done at least 3–6 months before conception attempts and discontinued once actively trying to conceive. Mobilizing toxins during pregnancy is not recommended.

Clinical Pearl: Support all detoxification efforts with adequate hydration (typically half your body weight in ounces of filtered water daily), fiber intake (at least 35g daily), and regular exercise to stimulate lymphatic flow.

NUTRITIONAL ARCHITECTURE

Blueprint-Specific Nutrition: Eating for Hormonal Balance

Beyond general fertility nutrition, specific hormonal imbalances benefit from targeted nutritional strategies:

Estrogen Dominance Pattern

If you have symptoms of excess estrogen relative to progesterone (heavy periods, breast tenderness, fibroids, endometriosis, PMS):

- **Dietary Focus:**
    - Cruciferous vegetables daily (broccoli, cauliflower, kale, Brussels sprouts)
    - Ground flaxseeds (2 tablespoons daily)
    - Adequate fiber (at least 35g daily) to support estrogen elimination
    - Reduce alcohol, which impairs estrogen metabolism
    - Choose organic animal products to avoid added hormones

- **Supplements to Consider:**
    - Diindolylmethane (DIM)
    - Calcium D-glucarate
    - Curcumin
    - Rosemary extract

Low Progesterone Pattern

If you have signs of insufficient progesterone (short luteal phase, spotting before periods, anxiety, sleep disruption):

- **Dietary Focus:**
    - Emphasize zinc-rich foods (oysters, pumpkin seeds, grass-fed beef)

- Include vitamin C-rich foods (citrus, bell peppers, berries)
- Consume sufficient healthy cholesterol for hormone precursors
- Focus on B6-rich foods (wild salmon, sweet potatoes, pistachios)
- Reduce high-intensity exercise, which can lower progesterone

- **Supplements to Consider:**
  - Vitex (chasteberry)
  - Vitamin B6
  - Magnesium
  - Vitamin C

Insulin Resistance Pattern

If you have PCOS, metabolic syndrome, or other signs of insulin resistance:

- **Dietary Focus:**
  - Lower carbohydrate approach (typically 15–30% of calories)
  - Emphasize protein with each meal (at least 30g per meal)
  - Include insulin-sensitizing spices (cinnamon, turmeric, ginger)
  - Consider intermittent fasting if appropriate (16:8 method often works well)
  - Eliminate all refined sugars and flours

- **Supplements to Consider:**
    - Inositol (myo-inositol and D-chiro-inositol in 40:1 ratio)
    - Berberine
    - Alpha-lipoic acid
    - Chromium
    - N-acetyl cysteine (NAC)

Thyroid Support Pattern

If you have hypothyroidism or subclinical thyroid dysfunction:

- **Dietary Focus:**
    - Include iodine-rich foods if appropriate (seaweed, fish, eggs)
    - Ensure sufficient selenium (Brazil nuts, sardines, grass-fed beef)
    - Minimize raw cruciferous vegetables, which can be goitrogenic
    - Eliminate gluten, which can cross-react with thyroid tissue
    - Support zinc and copper balance for T4 to T3 conversion

- **Supplements to Consider:**
    - Selenium
    - Zinc
    - Iron (if ferritin is low)
    - Tyrosine
    - Ashwagandha

Clinical Pearl: Nutritional approaches should be adapted throughout your menstrual cycle. In general, the follicular phase benefits from higher carbohydrate intake and lighter foods, while the luteal phase benefits from higher protein and fat intake with warming, grounding foods.

NATURAL BUILDING MATERIALS: HERBAL THERAPIES FOR FERTILITY

Herbs have been used to support reproductive health for thousands of years. Modern research is now validating many traditional applications. These natural building materials can provide gentle yet effective support for your fertility blueprint:

Female Fertility Herbs
- **Vitex (Chasteberry):**
    - **Actions:** Supports pituitary function, improves progesterone production, regulates cycles
    - **Best For:** Luteal phase defects, irregular cycles, PMS
    - **Usage:** Most effective when used consistently for at least 3–6 months
    - **Caution:** May not be appropriate for those with high prolactin

- **Shatavari (Asparagus racemosus):**
    - **Actions:** Phytoestrogenic, supports follicular development, improves cervical mucus
    - **Best For:** Dry cervical mucus, estrogen deficiency, reproductive tonification
    - **Usage:** Can be used as tea, tincture, or capsules
    - **Synergy:** Combines well with licorice for hormone balance

- **Red Clover (Trifolium pratense):**
  - **Actions:** Contains isoflavones that gently support estrogen function
  - **Best For:** Improving cervical mucus, supporting estrogen in perimenopause
  - **Usage:** Often used as tea or tincture
  - **Research:** Shows benefits for endometrial health

- **Maca (Lepidium meyenii):**
  - **Actions:** Adaptogenic, supports hormone production, enhances libido
  - **Best For:** Stress-related fertility issues, hypothalamic amenorrhea, low libido
  - **Usage:** Gelatinized form is more digestible; typically used as powder
  - **Note:** Works gradually over time, not immediately

Male Fertility Herbs

- **Ashwagandha (Withania somnifera):**
  - **Actions:** Reduces stress hormones, supports testosterone production, improves sperm parameters
  - **Best For:** Stress-related fertility issues, low testosterone, poor sperm quality
  - **Usage:** Most studied at 600mg daily
  - **Research:** Multiple studies show improvements in sperm count and motility

- **Tribulus (Tribulus terrestris):**
  - **Actions:** Supports testosterone production, improves erectile function

- Best For: Low libido, mild erectile dysfunction, low sperm count
- Usage: Standardized to contain 45% saponins
- Caution: May increase DHT; avoid with DHT-sensitive conditions

- **Pine Pollen:**
  - **Actions:** Contains natural androgens, supports testosterone
  - **Best For:** Low testosterone, fatigue, reduced sperm quality
  - **Usage:** Available as powder or tincture
  - **Note:** Tincture has stronger hormonal effects than powder

General Reproductive Tonics
- **Dong Quai (Angelica sinensis):**
  - **Actions:** Improves circulation to reproductive organs, blood building
  - **Best For:** Blood stagnation, poor uterine blood flow, anemia
  - **Caution:** Avoid during heavy menstruation or pregnancy

- **Schisandra (Schisandra chinensis):**
  - **Actions:** Adaptogenic, liver supporting, antioxidant
  - **Best For:** Stress-related infertility, poor egg quality, liver congestion
  - **Usage:** Can be used as berry, powder, or tincture

- **Raspberry Leaf (Rubus idaeus):**
  - **Actions:** Tones uterine tissue, rich in fertility nutrients
  - **Best For:** General uterine health, preparation for pregnancy
  - **Usage:** Often used as tea, 1–3 cups daily

Important Note: Herbal therapy should be personalized based on your specific constitution and fertility challenges. Work with a practitioner trained in herbal medicine for the best results, especially when combining herbs with fertility medications.

CHAPTER 20

BODY WORK AND ENERGY SYSTEMS

CHIROPRACTIC CARE: OPTIMIZING YOUR BODY'S STRUCTURAL FOUNDATION FOR FERTILITY

In our home renovation metaphor, chiropractic care functions as structural engineering for your body's framework—ensuring that the foundation and support systems are properly aligned to allow optimal function of all internal systems, including reproduction. Just as a house with a compromised frame can't support its electrical and plumbing systems effectively, spinal misalignments can interfere with the nervous system's ability to regulate reproductive function. I discuss this thoroughly in chapter 2 of *Your Longevity Blueprint*.

THE SPINE-FERTILITY CONNECTION

Our vertebrae protect our spinal cord, and our skull protects our brain—the command centers that control every aspect of reproductive function. The framework of a home is slightly flexible, designed to give and

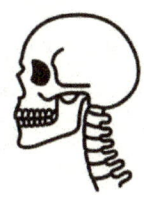

take with environmental stresses. Have you ever been in a high-rise building and felt it moving with the wind? The architect allowed for that flexibility. The same holds true for the spine.

The spine is made of several vertebrae, which can tolerate some movement and adjustment. While a mild curvature of the spine doesn't typically cause major problems, these misalignments should be corrected for optimal function of our bodies—especially when we're trying to optimize something as delicate as reproductive health.

Your nervous system controls blood flow to organs for them to function properly, and if blood flow or nerve impulses are impaired, you can end up with pain or even lowered organ function. This principle is particularly crucial for fertility, where optimal nerve communication and blood flow to reproductive organs can make the difference between conception and continued struggle.

HOW SPINAL ALIGNMENT AFFECTS REPRODUCTIVE FUNCTION

Nervous System Communication: The nerves that control reproductive organs originate from specific areas of the spine:

- **Lumbar spine (L1–L2):** Nerves that supply the ovaries and uterine function
- **Sacral spine (S2–S4):** Nerves controlling uterine contractions and pelvic floor function
- **Upper cervical spine:** Houses the connection between brain and reproductive hormone centers

When these vertebrae are misaligned, nerve interference can disrupt the precise communication needed for:

- Proper hormone production and regulation
- Optimal blood flow to reproductive organs

- Coordination between the brain and reproductive system
- Healthy pelvic floor function supporting implantation

Blood Flow Optimization: Spinal alignment directly affects circulation throughout the body. Proper alignment ensures:
- Adequate blood flow to ovaries for healthy egg development
- Optimal uterine blood flow for endometrial development and implantation
- Proper circulation to support the entire reproductive system
- Enhanced lymphatic drainage to reduce inflammation in reproductive tissues

Stress Response Regulation: The spine houses the nervous system pathways that control our stress response. Proper alignment supports:
- Balanced sympathetic and parasympathetic nervous system function
- Improved stress hormone regulation (crucial for fertility)
- Better sleep quality (essential for hormone production)
- Enhanced overall nervous system resilience

PERSONAL CONNECTION TO STRUCTURAL HEALTH

I was raised in a family that always went to the chiropractor to assess our body's framework and make sure our spines were restored to proper alignment, and we really never became sick. This early understanding of the body's structural foundation has informed my approach to fertility care throughout my career.

I have continued seeing a chiropractor my entire life, and especially throughout my fertility journey. During those ten years of trying to conceive, regular chiropractic care was one of the consistent supports I maintained. While I was addressing hormonal imbalances, nutritional deficiencies, and environmental toxins, I also recognized that my body's structural foundation needed to be optimized to support the complex process of reproduction.

My chiropractors helped me understand that pain or dysfunction frequently stems from compressed nerves in the spine or from muscle adhesions that create tension in surrounding areas. When they adjust a restricted joint back into proper alignment, it releases pressure on the affected nerve and allows normal function to return.

This principle applies beautifully to fertility challenges—sometimes the "dysfunction" isn't in the reproductive organs themselves, but in the structural framework that supports their optimal function. Throughout my own fertility struggles, I found that maintaining proper spinal alignment was an essential component of my comprehensive approach.

CHIROPRACTIC APPROACHES FOR FERTILITY SUPPORT
General Spinal Health
- **Full spine assessment** to identify areas of restriction or misalignment
- **Regular adjustments** to maintain optimal nervous system function
- **Postural corrections** to support overall structural integrity
- **Movement education** to maintain spinal health between visits

Fertility-Specific Techniques
- **Webster Technique:** Specifically designed to optimize pelvic alignment and reduce intrauterine constraint
- **Sacral adjustments:** To ensure proper nerve function to reproductive organs
- **Thoracic spine care:** Supporting the nerves that affect circulation and breathing
- **Upper cervical work:** Optimizing brain-body communication for hormone regulation

Supportive Therapies
- **Soft tissue work** to address muscle tension that may affect spinal alignment
- **Pelvic floor coordination** exercises and education
- **Breathing techniques** that support both spinal health and stress management
- **Ergonomic counseling** for work and daily activities

Integration with Other Fertility Therapies
Chiropractic care enhances other fertility interventions by:
- **Supporting Acupuncture:** Proper spinal alignment can enhance the effectiveness of acupuncture treatments by improving nerve conduction and energy flow throughout the body.
- **Enhancing Nutritional Therapy:** Better nervous system function supports improved digestion, nutrient absorption, and hormone metabolism.
- **Amplifying Stress Reduction:** A properly aligned spine supports better stress hormone regulation and nervous system resilience.

- **Optimizing Medical Treatments:** Whether pursuing natural conception or assisted reproductive technologies, optimal structural health supports the best possible outcomes.

FINDING THE RIGHT CHIROPRACTOR FOR FERTILITY SUPPORT
Look for practitioners with:
- Experience working with fertility patients
- Understanding of the reproductive system and hormonal health
- Training in fertility-specific techniques like the Webster Technique
- Collaborative approach with other healthcare providers
- Gentle techniques appropriate for women trying to conceive

Red flags to avoid:
- Aggressive adjustment techniques that create more stress
- Practitioners who dismiss the mind-body connection
- Those who promise unrealistic outcomes
- Lack of understanding about fertility challenges and sensitivities

TREATMENT TIMELINE AND EXPECTATIONS
Initial Phase (Weeks 1–4):
- Comprehensive assessment and initial corrections
- Most acute misalignments addressed
- Beginning of improved nervous system function

Optimization Phase (Weeks 4–12):
- Regular maintenance adjustments
- Structural patterns become more stable
- Nervous system function continues to improve

Maintenance Phase (Ongoing):
- Regular check-ups to maintain alignment
- Proactive care to prevent regression
- Continued support throughout conception attempts and pregnancy

Just as you wouldn't attempt to renovate a house with a compromised foundation, optimizing your fertility requires ensuring that your body's structural framework can support the complex processes of reproduction. Chiropractic care provides this essential foundation, creating the optimal environment for your body's natural fertility to flourish.

The beauty of chiropractic care in fertility support is that it works with your body's innate wisdom rather than against it—removing interference so your reproductive system can function as it was designed to. When combined with the other elements of your fertility blueprint, proper structural alignment becomes another powerful tool in creating the optimal conditions for new life.

ACUPUNCTURE: ANCIENT WISDOM FOR MODERN FERTILITY

In our home renovation metaphor, acupuncture functions as a sophisticated energy system optimization—similar to how an electrician might restore proper current flow throughout your home's wiring. This ancient practice, with over 3,000 years

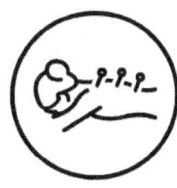

of history, works by stimulating specific points on the body to balance the flow of qi (pronounced "chee"), or vital energy, through pathways called meridians.

THE FERTILITY-ACUPUNCTURE CONNECTION

Modern research increasingly validates what Traditional Chinese Medicine (TCM) has understood for millennia: proper energy flow is essential for reproductive function. When applied to fertility, acupuncture offers several evidence-based benefits:

Hormonal Regulation:
- Stimulates the hypothalamic-pituitary-ovarian axis to improve hormone production and regulation
- Helps normalize irregular cycles by enhancing communication between the brain and reproductive organs
- Supports ovulation by improving follicular development and maturation
- May reduce elevated androgens in conditions like PCOS

Blood Flow Enhancement:
- Increases blood flow to the uterus and ovaries by up to 15-20%, according to research
- Improves endometrial thickness and receptivity
- Enhances oxygen and nutrient delivery to reproductive tissues
- Supports implantation by creating an optimal endometrial environment

Stress Reduction:
- Triggers release of endorphins, the body's natural stress-relievers
- Reduces cortisol levels that can interfere with reproductive hormones
- Activates the parasympathetic ("rest and digest") nervous system
- Improves sleep quality, which is essential for hormone production

Inflammation Modulation:
- Helps reduce systemic and localized inflammation
- May benefit inflammatory conditions like endometriosis
- Supports proper immune function at the implantation site
- Helps balance the body's inflammatory response

MY PERSONAL EXPERIENCE WITH ACUPUNCTURE

Acupuncture played a significant role in my own fertility journey. Between unsuccessful fertility treatments and before conceiving my son Michael, I integrated regular acupuncture sessions into my comprehensive protocol. The treatments not only supported my reproductive system but also provided much-needed stress relief during an emotionally challenging time.

What surprised me most was how individualized the treatments were—my acupuncturist adjusted the protocol based on where I was in my cycle, my specific symptoms, and the underlying patterns she identified. I received acupuncture post ovulation and post transfer to help with implantation. This personalized approach perfectly complemented the functional medicine work I was doing simultaneously.

RESEARCH-BACKED BENEFITS FOR FERTILITY

The scientific evidence for acupuncture's benefits in fertility continues to grow:

- 2020 randomized controlled clinic trials have shown sessions of acupuncture before and after embryo transfer significantly increased the pregnancy rates in women with unexplained infertility.[5]
- Studies show acupuncture can increase sperm count, motility, and quality in male fertility cases.
- A landmark study at Reproductive Medicine and Fertility Center in Colorado found that combining acupuncture with IVF led to a 26% higher pregnancy rate.[6]

PRACTICAL IMPLEMENTATION

When to Consider Acupuncture:

- At any point in your fertility journey, even while preparing for conception
- Particularly beneficial with hormonal imbalances like irregular cycles or luteal phase defects
- During fertility treatment cycles (IUI or IVF) to enhance outcomes
- When stress is a significant factor in your fertility challenges
- In cases of unexplained infertility

---

5   Zhou, X., Li, X., Ding, H., Lu, Y. (2023). Effects of acupuncture on pregnancy outcomes in women undergoing in vitro fertilization: an updated systematic review and meta-analysis. *Archives of Gynecology and Obstetrics*, 308(1), 179-192.

6   Dieterle, S., Li, C., Greb, R., Bartzsch, F., Hatzmann, W., Huang, D. (2009). A rospective randomized placebo-controlled study of the effect of acupuncture in infertile patients with severe oligoasthenozoospermia. *Fertility and Sterility*, 92(2), 572-574.

Finding the Right Practitioner:
- Look for certification by the National Certification Commission for Acupuncture and Oriental Medicine (NCCAOM)
- Seek practitioners who specialize in fertility and reproductive health
- Consider those with specialized training through organizations like the American Board of Oriental Reproductive Medicine (ABORM)
- Ask about their experience with your specific fertility challenge

Optimal Treatment Timeline:
- For general fertility support: weekly sessions for at least 3 months
- For cycle regulation: begin with twice weekly for 1 month, then reassess
- For IVF support: sessions during stimulation phase, plus treatments before and after embryo transfer
- For male factor: twice weekly for at least 2–3 months to align with sperm development cycle

What to Expect During Treatment:
- A comprehensive intake examining your entire health history, not just fertility factors
- Pulse and tongue diagnosis (common TCM diagnostic methods)
- Very thin needles placed at specific points (typically painless or with minimal sensation)

- A typical session lasts 30–60 minutes, often with time for the needles to remain in place
- You may receive additional recommendations for herbs, dietary changes, or lifestyle modifications

INTEGRATION WITH FUNCTIONAL MEDICINE

Acupuncture and functional medicine complement each other beautifully in addressing fertility challenges:

- Both view the body as an interconnected system rather than isolated parts
- Each recognizes the importance of individualized treatment
- Both address the underlying patterns and root causes, not just symptoms
- Acupuncture can help reduce side effects from fertility medications while enhancing their effectiveness
- The stress-reduction benefits of acupuncture support the hormonal balance work of functional medicine

For optimal results, share your functional medicine test results and treatment plans with your acupuncturist, and likewise, share your acupuncture experiences with your functional medicine practitioner. This integrative approach creates a powerful synergy that addresses fertility challenges from multiple angles simultaneously.

Just as a comprehensive home renovation benefits from both modern structural engineers and craftspeople skilled in traditional building arts, your fertility renovation can be enhanced by combining modern functional medicine with the ancient wisdom of acupuncture—creating balance from both the biochemical and energetic perspectives.

CHAPTER 21

IMPLEMENTATION AND PROFESSIONAL SUPPORT

In our home renovation metaphor, this chapter serves as your comprehensive project management guide and contractor network directory—the essential blueprint for orchestrating your fertility renovation from initial planning through final completion. Just as a successful home renovation requires careful sequencing of trades (you can't install hardwood floors before the plumbing rough-in is complete), your fertility optimization follows a strategic timeline where foundational work must be established before advanced systems can be properly integrated. Like a seasoned general contractor who knows when to bring in specialized subcontractors—electricians for complex wiring, structural engineers for load-bearing modifications, or HVAC specialists for climate control—your fertility journey may require professional support at key intervals to ensure optimal results. This chapter provides your detailed implementation timeline and helps you identify when your

DIY efforts need reinforcement from fertility specialists, functional medicine practitioners, or other therapeutic professionals to complete your reproductive renovation successfully.

THE DIY TIMELINE: IMPLEMENTING YOUR FERTILITY RENOVATION

For optimal results, implement these DIY fertility improvements in a strategic sequence:

Months 1–2: Foundation Work
- Begin stress reduction practices daily
- Implement fertility nutrition plan
- Start basic supplements (prenatal, omega-3, CoQ10)
- Remove obvious toxins from environment and personal care
- Begin gentle detoxification support
- Establish fertility tracking methods

Months 3–4: Systems Optimization
- Add targeted supplements based on testing results
- Implement specific herbal protocols if indicated
- Intensify detoxification if needed
- Refine stress management techniques
- Begin specialized therapies if required (under practitioner guidance)
- Continue refined nutrition plan

Months 5–6: Fine-Tuning and Integration
- Adjust protocols based on observed changes
- Optimize cycle-specific strategies
- Integrate conventional fertility treatments if needed
- Maintain core stress management and nutrition

- Begin active conception attempts if all systems are optimized
- Transition from detoxification to maintenance

Remember that the eggs and sperm being released today began their developmental journey 3–4 months ago. This means the improvements you implement now will benefit the eggs and sperm that will be ready 3–4 months from now. This biological timeline explains why patience and consistency are so important in fertility optimization.

> **Success Story:** After three years of unexplained infertility and two failed IVF cycles, Caroline and Michael decided to take six months to fully implement a comprehensive DIY fertility protocol before their final IVF attempt. They eliminated inflammatory foods, optimized their sleep, practiced daily stress reduction, removed all toxins from their home environment, implemented targeted supplementation based on testing, and followed personalized herbal protocols. When they returned for their third IVF cycle, their doctor was amazed—Caroline produced 14 high-quality eggs (compared to 6 poor-quality eggs in her previous cycle), and Michael's sperm parameters had improved dramatically. They used acupuncture post transfer and achieved pregnancy with their first embryo transfer and now have a healthy daughter.

SPECIALIZED CONSTRUCTION TECHNIQUES: THERAPEUTIC SUPPORT

In some cases, specialized interventions may be necessary to support your fertility renovation. These approaches should be implemented under professional guidance but are important to understand as potential options in your fertility toolkit.

FRAMEWORK SUPPORT: HCG INJECTIONS

Human Chorionic Gonadotropin (hCG) is a hormone naturally produced during pregnancy, but it can also be used therapeutically to support fertility:

- **Mechanism of Action:**
    - Mimics luteinizing hormone (LH)
    - Stimulates ovulation in women
    - Increases testosterone production in men
    - Supports luteal phase function

- **Fertility Applications:**
    - **Trigger Shot:** Used to precisely time ovulation in medicated cycles
    - **Luteal Phase Support:** Low-dose hCG can support corpus luteum function
    - **Male Fertility Enhancement:** Can stimulate testosterone and sperm production
    - **Hypothalamic Amenorrhea:** May help restart ovulation in some cases

- **Administration:**
    - Typically given as injection (subcutaneous or intramuscular)
    - Dosing varies widely based on purpose

- o Timing is crucial for effectiveness
- o Requires prescription and medical supervision

- **Considerations:**
  - o Not appropriate for all fertility situations
  - o May cause ovarian hyperstimulation in sensitive individuals
  - o Monitoring is essential when using for ovulation induction
  - o Often combined with other fertility medications

STRUCTURAL REINFORCEMENT: PROGESTERONE THERAPY

Progesterone is essential for implantation and pregnancy maintenance. Supplemental progesterone can provide crucial support in cases of deficiency:

- **Types of Progesterone:**
  - o **Bioidentical:** Molecularly identical to human progesterone
  - o **Synthetic:** Progestins like medroxyprogesterone acetate (less recommended for fertility)

- **Delivery Methods:**
  - o **Vaginal:** Suppositories, gels, or tablets placed vaginally (preferred for fertility)
  - o **Oral:** Capsules taken by mouth (undergoes liver metabolism)
  - o **Injectable:** Oil-based injections (highest blood levels, used in specific protocols)

- o **Transdermal:** Creams applied to skin (may not provide sufficient levels for fertility support)

- **Fertility Applications:**
    - o **Luteal Phase Support:** Correcting short luteal phase or inadequate progesterone production
    - o **Post-Ovulation Supplementation:** Supporting implantation and early pregnancy
    - o **Recurrent Pregnancy Loss:** Preventing miscarriage in progesterone-deficient individuals
    - o **After Fertility Treatments:** Supporting pregnancies after IUI or IVF

- **Timing Considerations:**
    - o Typically started after confirmed ovulation
    - o Often continued until 10–12 weeks of pregnancy if conception occurs
    - o Abrupt discontinuation during early pregnancy can increase miscarriage risk

- **Monitoring Recommendations:**
    - o Progesterone levels should be checked before supplementation
    - o Follow-up testing may be warranted to ensure adequate levels
    - o Ultrasounds may be recommended to confirm ongoing pregnancy development

Clinical Pearl: The combination of lifestyle changes, nutritional support, and targeted natural interventions often reduces or eliminates the need for more intensive medical interventions. However, when specialized support like hCG or progesterone is needed, integrating it with a comprehensive functional approach typically yields the best results.

LOW DOSE NALTREXONE: ADVANCED INFLAMMATION CONTROL SYSTEM

Within our home renovation metaphor, Low Dose Naltrexone (LDN) functions like an advanced climate control system that regulates the internal environment of your reproductive home—specifically targeting excess inflammation and immune dysregulation that can compromise fertility across numerous conditions.

Understanding LDN's Mechanism

Naltrexone was originally developed as an opioid antagonist at high doses (50mg), but when used at much lower doses (typically 1.5–4.5mg), it creates a completely different effect:

1. **Inflammation Reduction:**
    - LDN temporarily blocks endorphin receptors during nighttime hours, triggering your body to produce more endorphins and enkephalins
    - These natural compounds help regulate the immune system and reduce inflammatory cytokines
    - The result is a dampening of the excessive inflammation that contributes to many fertility challenges

2. **Immune System Modulation:**
    - LDN helps balance overactive immune responses that may attack reproductive tissues
    - For conditions with autoimmune components (like some cases of endometriosis, unexplained infertility, and

recurrent pregnancy loss), LDN helps restore proper immune tolerance
- This is particularly valuable for implantation success, where immune rejection of an embryo can occur

3. **Endorphin Optimization:**
   - Higher endorphin levels improve overall pain management
   - Better endorphin function supports healthy stress response and sleep quality
   - Enhanced mood and reduced anxiety can further support fertility

LDN APPLICATIONS ACROSS FERTILITY CHALLENGES

This versatile tool can provide support for multiple fertility obstacles:

1. **Endometriosis:** Reduces the inflammatory cascade that drives lesion development and pain
2. **PCOS:** Improves insulin sensitivity and may help regulate cycles
3. **Unexplained Infertility:** Addresses potential undiagnosed immune or inflammatory factors
4. **Recurrent Pregnancy Loss:** Modulates immune factors that may reject embryos
5. **Thyroid Autoimmunity:** Helps reduce antibody production in Hashimoto's thyroiditis
6. **Inflammatory Male Factor Issues:** May improve sperm parameters by reducing systemic inflammation

MY PERSONAL EXPERIENCE WITH LDN

LDN played a significant role in my own fertility journey. After discovering multiple underlying conditions—including endometriosis, subtle immune dysfunction, and persistent inflammation—I added LDN to my comprehensive protocol years before conceiving my son Michael. While it wasn't the only intervention I used, I believe it significantly contributed to creating a more receptive environment for pregnancy by addressing the underlying inflammatory and immune components of my fertility challenges.

The beauty of LDN is that it works with your body's own regulatory systems rather than overriding them, similar to a smart thermostat that makes subtle adjustments to maintain optimal conditions rather than forcing dramatic temperature swings.

Practical Implementation

When considering LDN as part of your fertility renovation:

1. **Professional Guidance:**
   - LDN requires a prescription and should be used under medical supervision
   - Work with a provider experienced in LDN for fertility applications
   - Ideal dosing varies by individual and condition
2. **Timing Considerations:**
   - Typically taken at bedtime due to its effects on endorphin release during sleep
   - Best results occur after 3–6 months of consistent use
   - Can be continued during IVF cycles and often through the pregnancy (with provider approval) but needs to be stopped by 36 weeks

3. **Formulation Matters:**
    - Must be compounded by a pharmacy experienced with LDN
    - Avoid fillers like lactose or slow-release formulations
    - Available as capsules, liquid, or sublingual formulations
4. **Potential Adjustments:**
    - Some individuals need to start at very low doses (0.5mg) and gradually increase
    - Temporary sleep disturbances may occur when starting and typically resolve within weeks
    - Occasional vivid dreams are reported as endorphin production increases

As with any specialized construction technique, LDN is not a standalone solution but rather an integrated component of a comprehensive approach to fertility optimization. When combined with proper nutrition, stress management, hormone balancing, and addressing specific structural issues, LDN can enhance your body's natural capacity for healing and reproductive function.

PARTNERING WITH PROFESSIONALS: WHEN TO SEEK HELP

While many fertility improvements can be implemented on your own, certain situations warrant professional guidance:

- **When to Consult a Functional Medicine Practitioner:**
    - If you've been trying to conceive for over 6 months (over age 35) or 12 months (under age 35)
    - When basic interventions haven't produced cycle improvements after 3 months
    - If you have known health conditions affecting fertility

- When you need comprehensive hormone or other specialized testing
- For personalized protocols based on your specific health history
- To safely integrate natural approaches with conventional fertility treatments

- **When to See a Reproductive Endocrinologist:**
  - If you're over age 35 and have been trying for 6+ months
  - If you're over age 40 (consider immediate consultation)
  - When known structural issues exist (blocked tubes, severe endometriosis, etc.)
  - If you have a history of recurrent pregnancy loss
  - When male factor infertility is severe
  - If time is a significant concern

Remember that DIY fertility improvements and medical treatments are not mutually exclusive. The most successful fertility journeys often combine the best of both approaches—using functional medicine to create the optimal internal environment while utilizing appropriate medical technologies when needed.

By implementing these DIY fertility improvements, you're not just passively waiting for conception to occur—**you're actively creating the ideal conditions for new life to begin.** Like a homeowner who takes pride in preparing their space before professional renovations, you're doing the essential groundwork that will enhance the effectiveness of any additional fertility treatments you might need.

In the next section, we'll conclude our fertility blueprint by examining what happens when all these elements come together successfully—looking at real-life renovation success stories and planning for your future family.

YOUR LONGEVITY BLUEPRINT NUTRACEUTICAL PRODUCTS

Here are my favorite Your Longevity Blueprint products to address needs mentioned in this section:

- Adrenal Calm
- Alpha Lipoic Acid
- Berberine Support
- GI Support
- Gut Shield
- Herbal Adrenal Complex
- Inositol Complex
- Iron Chelate
- Magnesium Chelate
- Methyl B complex
- NAC
- Omega 3s
- SL Methyl Bs
- Zinc Chelate

You can download product data sheets with details on each of these products at yourlongevityblueprint.com, and use the code "fertility" for 10% off.

SECTION VI

CONCLUSION—THE COMPLETED PROJECT

CHAPTER 22

SUCCESS STORIES AND FUTURE PLANNING

Throughout this book, we've explored the complex process of renovating your reproductive home—addressing everything from the foundation and framework to the heating and cooling system, specialized rooms, and finishing touches. Just as a home renovation transforms a structure into a welcoming space for living, the fertility renovation process transforms your body into a nurturing environment for new life.

We've examined the science behind functional medicine approaches to fertility, explored the interconnectedness of body systems, and provided practical strategies for optimizing your reproductive health. Now it's time to look at what happens when all these elements come together successfully—when the renovation is complete and the home is ready for its new occupant.

MODEL HOMES: SUCCESS STORIES FROM PATIENTS

Throughout this book, I've shared various patient success stories, each highlighting different aspects of the fertility renovation process. These "model homes" demonstrate the principles in action and provide inspiration for your own fertility journey. Let me share a few more stories that illustrate the power of the functional medicine approach:

HANNAH AND DAVID: THE FOUNDATION RENOVATION

Hannah and David came to me after three years of unexplained infertility. Standard testing showed nothing obviously wrong—Hannah was ovulating, David's sperm parameters were normal, and Hannah's tubes were open. Yet month after month, they failed to conceive.

Comprehensive functional testing revealed significant gut dysbiosis in both partners, with Hannah showing high levels of intestinal permeability ("leaky gut"). This foundation issue was creating systemic inflammation that affected hormone signaling and egg quality. Additionally, David's semen analysis showed high levels of oxidative stress not detected in standard testing.

Their renovation plan focused on:
- A 60-day gut healing protocol for both partners
- Elimination of inflammatory foods, particularly gluten and dairy
- Targeted antioxidant support for sperm health
- Stress reduction techniques to address elevated cortisol levels

After four months on this protocol, Hannah's inflammatory markers normalized, and David's semen analysis showed significant improvements in sperm DNA integrity. They conceived naturally in their fifth month and now have a healthy baby boy.

Their story demonstrates how addressing the foundation—gut health and inflammation—can resolve seemingly unexplained fertility challenges.

MELISSA: THE ELECTRICAL SYSTEM REWIRING

Melissa, a 34-year-old attorney, came to me with regular cycles but severe PMS, anxiety, and two early miscarriages. Her conventional doctor had suggested trying again and considering IVF if she experienced a third loss.

Our testing revealed a classic case of electrical system dysfunction—HPA axis dysregulation with elevated evening cortisol and depleted morning cortisol, along with low progesterone during the luteal phase. Essentially, her body's stress response system was sending improper signals to her reproductive system.

Her renovation plan included:
- Targeted adaptogenic herbs to regulate the HPA axis
- Heart rate variability training to improve autonomic nervous system function
- Significant work schedule modifications to reduce stress exposure
- Natural progesterone support during the luteal phase
- Magnesium and B vitamin repletion

Within three months, Melissa's cortisol rhythm normalized, her PMS symptoms reduced by 80%, and her luteal phase progesterone levels doubled. She conceived in her fourth month and, with continued progesterone support, carried to term without complications.

Her case illustrates how rewiring the electrical system—the stress response and communication networks—can create a more hospitable environment for conception and pregnancy.

REBEKAH AND JAMES: THE ALTERNATIVE BLUEPRINT

Rebekah and James came to me seeking support for their surrogacy journey. They had selected an egg donor and surrogate but wanted to ensure the best possible outcome by optimizing the health of their sperm for the IVF process.

Comprehensive testing revealed suboptimal sperm parameters for James— along with high DNA fragmentation and low morphology. We implemented a three-month sperm optimization protocol:

- Targeted antioxidant therapy (CoQ10, vitamin C, vitamin E)
- Environmental toxin reduction in their home and workplace
- Cold therapy for the testicular area
- Stress management techniques
- Nutritional support focused on zinc, selenium, and omega-3 fatty acids

James showed significant improvements in sperm quality. When the time came for the IVF cycle, they were able to create multiple high-quality embryos. Their surrogate successfully carried and delivered a healthy baby girl.

Their story demonstrates that the functional approach applies to all family-building journeys, including those using assisted reproductive technologies and alternative family structures.

PLANNING YOUR FUTURE: RESOURCES FOR CONTINUED SUPPORT

The fertility renovation process doesn't end with conception—it continues through pregnancy, postpartum, and into the raising of your child. Here are resources to support you throughout this ongoing journey:

PROFESSIONAL SUPPORT NETWORKS

- **Finding a Functional Medicine Practitioner:** The Institute for Functional Medicine (IFM.org) and the American Academy of Anti-Aging Medicine (A4M) maintain directories of certified practitioners who can provide ongoing support. (A4M is who I completed my fellowship through in 2013).
- **Fertility-Focused Acupuncturists:** The American Board of Oriental Reproductive Medicine (ABORM.org) certifies acupuncturists specializing in fertility.
- **Reproductive Endocrinologists Open to Integrative Approaches:** The Society for Assisted Reproductive Technology (SART.org) can help you locate clinics in your area.
- **Mental Health Support:** Resolve (resolve.org) offers support groups and counselor referrals specializing in fertility and family building.

EDUCATIONAL RESOURCES

- **Books:**
    - *It Starts with the Egg* by Rebecca Fett
    - *The Fertility Diet* by Jorge Chavarro and Walter Willett
    - *Taking Charge of Your Fertility* by Toni Weschler
    - *Inconceivable* by Julia Indichova

- **Websites and Apps:**
    - Fertility Friend (fertilityfriend.com) for cycle tracking
    - Proov (proovtest.com) for at-home progesterone testing
    - Environmental Working Group (ewg.org) for toxin avoidance

- Mind/Body Fertility (mindandbodyfertility.com) for stress management resources

- **Courses and Programs:**
  - Fertility Awareness Method training
  - Mind/body fertility programs

ONGOING TESTING AND MONITORING
- Regular hormone testing to track improvements
- Nutritional status assessment every 6–12 months
- Microbiome testing annually
- Environmental toxin screening as needed

COMMUNITY CONNECTION
One of the most valuable resources on your fertility journey is connection with others who understand. Consider:
- Local or online support groups
- Fertility-focused yoga classes or meditation circles
- Community events for those building families
- Advocacy opportunities once your journey reaches its destination

MY TEN-YEAR JOURNEY: FROM HEARTBREAK TO HOPE

I need to be completely honest with you. Despite all my medical training, despite helping countless patients overcome their fertility challenges, despite knowing exactly what protocols to follow—it took me ten years to have my two children. Ten years.

Let that sink in for a moment. A provider who specializes in integrative medicine and hormone therapies, who had access to every test and treatment, who understood the science better than most—and I still struggled for a decade to build my family.

There were nights I cried myself to sleep, wondering if God had forgotten about me. There were moments I questioned everything I believed about healing and hope. There were days I wanted to give up on the dream of motherhood altogether.

The hardest part wasn't the physical challenges—though those were real. It wasn't even the failed treatments and disappointing test results. The hardest part was feeling like I should have had all the answers, and yet my own body seemed to be failing me despite everything I knew.

THE LESSONS ONLY STRUGGLE CAN TEACH

What I learned through those ten years of struggle has made me not just a better provider but a more compassionate human being. I learned that:

Knowledge alone isn't enough. Having all the right information doesn't guarantee the outcome you want. Sometimes God and the body have their own timeline that doesn't match our expectations or desires.

Persistence matters more than perfection. I made mistakes. I tried interventions that didn't work. I had to pivot and try new approaches multiple times. But I never gave up believing that God had children for Eric and me.

Faith and science aren't opposites—they're partners. My faith sustained me through the disappointments, while my medical knowledge guided my decisions. I needed both to navigate this journey successfully.

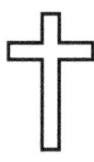

Every setback taught me something valuable. The failed IUIs taught me about timing. The endometriosis diagnosis taught me about hidden inflammation. The blood-clotting discoveries taught me about looking deeper when things don't make sense.

The journey changes you in ways the destination never could. By the time I held my sons, I was a completely different person—stronger, more empathetic, more grateful, and more equipped to help others facing similar struggles.

WHAT I DISCOVERED ALONG THE WAY

My personal fertility renovation ultimately required addressing multiple layers that I never would have uncovered without persistent investigation: the **inflammatory foods** (gluten and dairy) that were silently triggering immune responses. The **endocrine-disrupting chemicals** from hair straighteners and conventional products that I had unknowingly exposed myself to for years. The **chronic stress** patterns that had become so normal, I didn't recognize how they were affecting my hormones.

But the deeper discoveries came later. The **stage 4 endometriosis** that standard testing had missed. The **uterine inflammation** from chorioamnionitis that was preventing implantation. The **blood-clotting factors** that were compromising circulation to my reproductive organs.

Each discovery felt like finding another piece of a complex puzzle. Sometimes I felt overwhelmed by how many things needed to be addressed. But each piece we put in place brought me closer to my dream.

THE POWER OF NOT GIVING UP

Here's what I want you to understand: **I never actually needed IVF.** What I needed was proper diagnosis and treatment of the underlying conditions affecting my fertility. The IVF worked because we finally addressed the root causes—the inflammation, the infection, the blood flow issues.

But I almost gave up so many times. After my fourth failed IUI (I did eight total!), I wondered if I should just accept that biological children weren't meant for me…and then I got pregnant with William. After my third IVF transfer failed (I did seven total), I questioned whether I was being stubborn rather than faithful. I eventually conceived Michael.

What kept me going was my deep belief that God had a plan for our family. Even when I couldn't see it, even when the path seemed impossible, I held onto the promise that He would fulfill the desires of my heart in His perfect timing.

And He did. Both of my sons are miracles—not just because of the science that helped create them, but because of the journey of faith that brought them into existence.

I know what you might be thinking: "Wow, she did a lot to bring a baby into this world." And you're right—I did. Stress reduction, anti-inflammatory diet, countless supplements (especially antioxidants), IUIs, surgery, Clear Passage therapy, IVF, Mercier therapy, antibiotics, blood thinners, acupuncture, chiropractic care, and of course, prayer. The list goes on.

But I don't want this book to leave you thinking you have to do ALL of this. Think of me as the guinea pig who figured this out the long, hard way so that you don't have to. Every person's journey is different, and what worked for me might not be what your body needs.

The key is understanding the principles—addressing inflammation, supporting your body's natural systems, and finding the root causes—then working with qualified practitioners to determine which specific interventions make sense for your unique situation.

THE BROADER TRUTH ABOUT FERTILITY JOURNEYS

As we conclude this blueprint, I want to acknowledge that not all fertility renovations follow the expected timeline or result in a biological child. Some projects take unexpected turns, require different approaches, or lead to alternative forms of family building.

If you're reading this in the midst of your own struggle, please know that whatever path your renovation takes, the work you do to optimize your health through this functional medicine approach will benefit you throughout your lifetime. The improvements you make to your foundation, framework, and all the other components of your health "home" create a stronger structure for whatever the future holds.

Remember that a home is ultimately defined not by its physical features but by the love and connection it contains. Whether through biological conception, adoption, fostering, or choosing a child-free life full of meaning and purpose, your renovated health provides the perfect foundation for a fulfilling future.

WHAT I WANT YOU TO REMEMBER

After walking this path personally and professionally, here are the most important truths I want to leave with you:

Trust your intuition—it's often your first and best guide. I knew something wasn't right, that there was a root cause for IVF failing, and following that instinct led me to the answers that changed everything.

Your struggles don't define you—your persistence does. Every month that doesn't result in pregnancy isn't a failure; it's information. Every treatment that doesn't work isn't a dead end; it's redirection toward what will work.

Trust your instincts. If something doesn't feel right in your body, keep investigating. If a provider dismisses your concerns, find another provider. You know your body better than anyone else.

Address the whole system, not just the symptoms. The functional medicine approach in this book works because it recognizes that fertility is an expression of total body health, not just reproductive organ function.

Don't walk this journey alone. Whether it's your partner, family, friends, support groups, or healthcare providers—surround yourself with people who believe in your dream and will support you through the difficult times.

Hold onto hope, but release control. Do everything you can to optimize your health and fertility, then trust that the outcome will unfold as it's meant to. Sometimes the letting go is what allows the miracle to happen.

YOUR NEXT STEPS: BUILDING YOUR SUPPORT TEAM

Throughout this book, I've shared both the science behind fertility optimization and my personal journey to motherhood. While these pages contain a wealth of information to help you begin your own fertility renovation, I know from experience that personalized guidance can make all the difference in navigating this complex process.

At the Integrative Health and Hormone Clinic, my team and I pour our hearts into supporting everything discussed in this book. We understand the frustration, the hope, the disappointment, and the determination because we've walked similar paths ourselves. From detailed hormone testing and personalized supplement protocols to specialized fertility therapies and the emotional support that comes from working with practitioners who truly understand your journey—we're here to help you write your own success story.

If you're ready for personalized support on your fertility journey, we would be deeply honored to welcome you as a patient. Our clinic provides both in-person care at our Iowa location and virtual consultations for patients. Visit **ihhclinic.com** to learn more about our services and schedule your initial consultation. You can also **use the code "fertility" for 10% off** any products mentioned in this book at **yourlongevityblueprint.com**.

Remember that you don't have to walk this path alone. Whether you're just beginning to think about conception, have been struggling with fertility challenges for years, or are somewhere in between, our team is here to help you create your own miracle. Your fertility blueprint is unique—and with the right support, patience, and faith, you can build the family you've been dreaming of.

ONGOING EDUCATION AND SUPPORT THROUGH YOUR LONGEVITY BLUEPRINT PODCAST

Beyond personalized clinical care, I also invite you to join me each week on my podcast, also called Your Longevity Blueprint. On the show, we dive deeper into many of the concepts discussed in this book, and I share more of our personal health challenges and fertility struggles that didn't make it into these pages. Each episode explores the intricate interactions of nutrition, genetics, hormones, toxins, and infections using functional medicine principles to help you improve your health and longevity by finding the root cause of your symptoms.

Listen in each week to learn from experts at the top of their fields who share progressive, revolutionary, actionable tips, strategies, and resources to help you build your dream health from the ground up. Whether you're working on fertility optimization, hormone balance, or overall wellness, the podcast provides ongoing education and inspiration for your journey.

Please subscribe to the Your Longevity Blueprint podcast on all podcast platforms, and visit yourlongevityblueprint.com for additional resources and show notes. Consider it your weekly dose of hope and practical guidance as you continue building your fertility blueprint.

A FINAL REQUEST: SHARE THIS BLUEPRINT

Before I close, I have one important request. If this book has helped you, if the principles resonate with your heart, if you believe this approach could help others—please share it.

Share it with your sister who's just starting to think about having children. Share it with your friend who's been trying for months without success. Share it with your coworker who just had another disappointing fertility appointment. Share it with anyone who might benefit from understanding that there's another way—a comprehensive, hope-filled way—to approach fertility challenges.

So many people are suffering in silence, thinking their only options are "keep trying" or expensive medical procedures. They need to know about the power of addressing root causes. They need to know that their bodies have incredible healing capacity when given the right support. They need to know that they're not alone in this journey.

By sharing this blueprint, you're potentially changing someone's life. You're offering **hope** where there might be despair. You're providing answers where there might be confusion. You're extending the same gift of knowledge that I hope this book has given you.

WITH FAITH AND ENDLESS HOPE

As I write these final words, I'm looking at photos of my two miracle boys—William and Michael—and marveling at how God orchestrated every detail of their arrival. The ten-year journey that brought them to us wasn't the path I would have chosen, but it was exactly the path that prepared us to be their parents and me to write this book for you.

Your journey may look different from mine. It may be shorter or longer, simpler or more complex. But I believe with all my heart that if you don't give up, if you keep investigating, if you address your health holistically, and if you hold onto faith even in the darkest moments—your dream can become reality.

I'm praying for you. I'm believing for you. I'm cheering you on from Iowa as you begin or continue your own fertility renovation journey.

Don't give up. Your miracle may be just around the corner.

Wellness is Waiting™—and so is your family.

With love, hope, and endless faith in your journey,

Dr. Stephanie Gray

"For I know the plans I have for you," declares the LORD, "plans to prosper you and not to harm you, plans to give you hope and a future."
— Jeremiah 29:11

APPENDIX

FERTILITY BLUEPRINT RESOURCES

FERTILITY BLUEPRINT CHECKLIST

Use this comprehensive checklist to identify priority areas for your fertility renovation. Rate each area on a scale of 1–5:

    1 = Significant concern/symptoms
    3 = Moderate issues
    5 = Optimal function

FOUNDATION ASSESSMENT
DIGESTIVE SYSTEM

    ____ Regular, healthy bowel movements
    ____ Minimal gas, bloating or digestive discomfort
    ____ No food sensitivities or reactions
    ____ Appetite and digestion are balanced
    ____ No history of IBS, SIBO, or IBD
    ____ No use of antacids or digestive medications
    ____ Able to digest a wide variety of foods

Foundation Score: ____/35

DETOXIFICATION SYSTEM

    ____ Clear, healthy skin
    ____ No strong body odor
    ____ Minimal exposure to environmental toxins
    ____ Clean home environment (air, water, products)
    ____ Healthy liver function (normal lab values)
    ____ Regular, complete elimination
    ____ Clean personal care products
    ____ Limited alcohol consumption

Detoxification Score: ____/40

ELECTRICAL SYSTEM ASSESSMENT
NERVOUS SYSTEM

____ Adequate sleep (7–9 hours)

____ Ability to fall and stay asleep

____ Manageable stress levels

____ Mental clarity and focus

____ Stable mood and emotional balance

____ Ability to relax and wind down

____ Limited technology exposure at night

Electrical Score: ____/35

HEATING & COOLING ASSESSMENT
HORMONE BALANCE (WOMEN)

____ Regular menstrual cycles (26–35 days)

____ Minimal PMS symptoms

____ Normal flow (not too heavy or too light)

____ Minimal pain with menstruation

____ Stable energy throughout cycle

____ Healthy libido

____ Clear basal body temperature shift mid-cycle

____ Fertile-quality cervical mucus mid-cycle

____ No mid-cycle spotting

____ No luteal phase spotting

Female Hormone Score: ____/50

HORMONE BALANCE (MEN)
___ Healthy libido
___ Normal erectile function
___ Stable energy levels
___ Healthy body composition
___ Normal body hair distribution
___ Stable mood and motivation
___ Optimal sperm parameters (if tested)
___ No signs of testosterone deficiency
Male Hormone Score: ___/40

THYROID FUNCTION
___ Normal body temperature (97.8–98.6°F)
___ Stable energy throughout the day
___ Healthy hair, skin, and nails
___ Regular bowel movements
___ Appropriate weight for height
___ No cold hands and feet
___ Normal thyroid lab values
___ No thyroid medication required
Thyroid Score: ___/40

ADRENAL FUNCTION
___ Stable energy throughout the day
___ Appropriate stress response
___ Wake feeling refreshed
___ Handle stressful situations well
___ Normal blood pressure
___ No salt or sugar cravings
___ Healthy immune function
Adrenal Score: ___/35

PLUMBING SYSTEM ASSESSMENT
CIRCULATION & IMMUNE FUNCTION
____ Warm extremities
____ Normal clotting (not excessive)
____ Appropriate immune responses
____ Infrequent illnesses
____ No autoimmune conditions
____ Healthy inflammatory response
____ No chronic inflammatory conditions
____ Normal inflammatory markers on labs
____ No family history of blood clotting disorders

Plumbing Score: ____/45

STRUCTURAL INTEGRITY (FEMALE)
____ No pelvic pain
____ No pain with intercourse
____ No history of endometriosis
____ No history of PCOS
____ Normal reproductive anatomy
____ No fibroids or polyps
____ No ovarian cysts
____ No history of pelvic inflammatory disease
____ No history of STIs
____ No history of surgery on reproductive organs

Female Structure Score: ____/50

STRUCTURAL INTEGRITY (MALE)

____ No testicular pain or swelling

____ No varicocele

____ Normal ejaculatory function

____ No history of prostatitis

____ No history of STIs

____ No scrotal surgeries or trauma

____ No genital exposure to excessive heat

Male Structure Score: ____/35

ENVIRONMENTAL ASSESSMENT
ENVIRONMENTAL FACTORS

____ Limited EMF exposure

____ Clean water source

____ Organic food when possible

____ Limited processed food consumption

____ Air filtration in home

____ Limited occupational exposures

____ Limited use of plastics

____ Non-toxic household products

____ Limited alcohol consumption

____ No smoking or drug use

____ Limited caffeine consumption

Environment Score: ____/55

NUTRITIONAL STATUS

____ Adequate protein intake

____ Sufficient vegetable consumption

____ Healthy fat consumption

____ Limited sugar intake

____ Adequate hydration

____ Taking appropriate supplements

____ No nutritional deficiencies

____ Minimal processed food intake

____ Regular, balanced meals

Nutrition Score: ____/45

SCORING YOUR FERTILITY BLUEPRINT

Total all section scores: _____/460

PRIORITY DETERMINATION:

- Scores of 1–2 in any area indicate high-priority renovation needs
- Focus first on areas with lowest scores
- Address foundation issues before more specialized concerns

INTERPRETATION:

- **345–460**: Your fertility home is in excellent condition with only minor improvements needed
- **230–344**: Your fertility home needs moderate renovations in specific areas
- **115–229**: Your fertility home requires significant renovation in multiple systems
- **Below 115**: Your fertility home needs comprehensive reconstruction across all systems

NEXT STEPS

Based on your lowest-scoring areas, turn to the following chapters:
- Low Foundation Score: See Chapters 4, 17, and 19
- Low Electrical Score: See Chapters 7, 17, and 22
- Low Heating & Cooling Score: See Chapters 7-10 and 21
- Low Plumbing Score: See Chapters 7, 13, and 19
- Low Environmental Score: See Chapter 19 and 20

Remember that just as in home renovation, addressing foundation issues often improves other systems simultaneously. Focus on your lowest scores first, then progress to other areas as your health improves.

DOWNLOADABLE RESOURCES

For an updated list of all the supplements, tests, books, and products mentioned in this book, scan the QR code below or visit book landing page: www.yourfertilityblueprint.com.

Here you will also find free accompanying resources including:
- Testing Resources
- Fertility Supplement Protocols
- Fertility Meal Plan
- Fertility Renovation Timeline

Please note: Some links are affiliate links, which means I may earn a small commission if you purchase through them (at no extra cost to you). I only recommend products I personally use and trust, and the links offer special discounts to you.

ACKNOWLEDGMENTS

This book represents not only my personal journey but also the culmination of knowledge gained from exceptional educators, institutions, and colleagues who shaped my understanding of functional medicine and reproductive health.

I am deeply grateful to the American Academy of Anti-Aging Medicine (A4M), where I completed my fellowship in 2013. The comprehensive training in functional medicine principles provided me with the foundational tools I needed to look beyond symptoms and address root causes—an approach that proved essential not only for my patients but also for my own fertility journey. The education I received through A4M fundamentally changed how I practice medicine and ultimately made this book possible.

To the dedicated compounding pharmacists in my community who became invaluable teachers along the way—your willingness to share knowledge about bioidentical hormones, specialized formulations, and patient-specific treatments enriched my understanding immeasurably. Your expertise helped bridge the gap between functional medicine theory and practical application, benefiting countless patients over the years.

I extend sincere appreciation to Dr. Monica Minjeur, my primary care physician during my fertility journey, whose open-minded approach and collaborative spirit allowed me to integrate functional medicine principles with conventional care. Your willingness to work with me rather than against my holistic approach made all the difference.

My gratitude extends to the Pope Paul VI Institute, where Dr. Minjeur referred me for their groundbreaking work in reproductive medicine and natural fertility methods. It was at this institution that I underwent laparoscopic surgeries for endometriosis, a crucial step in my fertility journey. The research and clinical protocols developed by this institution provided crucial insights that influenced my approach to fertility optimization and helped me conceive my first son.

To the team at Clear Passage, whose innovative work addressing physical adhesions and structural barriers to fertility opened my eyes to the importance of physical therapy in reproductive health—your specialized techniques became an important piece of my own fertility puzzle.

I also acknowledge the University of Iowa's reproductive medicine program, where I ultimately received IVF treatment. The skilled physicians and staff who cared for me during this phase of my journey demonstrated how conventional and functional approaches can work together for optimal outcomes.

Finally, I must acknowledge my husband, Eric, who stood by me through every test, every treatment failure, every moment of doubt, and every small victory throughout our decade-long journey. While this book's Foreword speaks to his emotional support, here I must recognize his practical partnership—managing our clinic during my numerous appointments, supporting my continued education in functional medicine, and never questioning the time and resources invested in both my professional development and our fertility treatments. His unwavering belief in both my calling as a provider and our future as parents made this work possible.

Each of these individuals and institutions contributed essential knowledge, skills, or support that ultimately enabled me to write this book and help others on their fertility journeys. I am profoundly grateful for their contributions to both my professional development and personal healing.

REFERENCES

SECTION I
FERTILITY CRISIS STATISTICS

Levine et al. (2017) Temporal trends in sperm count: a systematic review and meta-regression analysis, *Human Reproduction Update*, 23(6), 646-659. (The landmark study showing 50% sperm decline.)

Practice Committee of American Society for Reproductive Medicine (2020) Definitions of infertility and recurrent pregnancy loss, *Fertility and Sterility*, 113(3), 533-535.

Sunderam et al. (2019) Assisted reproductive technology surveillance—United States, 2016, *MMWR Surveillance Summaries*, 68(4), 1-23.

World Health Organization (2023) Infertility Prevalence Estimates, 1990–2021, Global Health Observatory data.

ENVIRONMENTAL FACTORS

Gore et al. (2015) EDC-2: The Endocrine Society's second scientific statement on endocrine-disrupting chemicals, *Endocrine Reviews*, 36(6), E1-E150.

Ragusa et al. (2022) Placicenta: First evidence of microplastics in human placenta, *Environment International*, 146, 106274.

Swan et al. (2005) Decrease in anogenital distance among male infants with prenatal phthalate exposure, Environmental Health Perspectives, 113(8), 1056-1061.

FUNCTIONAL MEDICINE FOUNDATIONS

Bland, J. (2014) *The Disease Delusion: Conquering the Causes of Chronic Illness for a Healthier, Longer, and Happier Life*. HarperWave.

Gray, S. (2017) *Your Longevity Blueprint*, Avantage Media, Charleston, South Carolina.

Institute for Functional Medicine (2010) *Textbook of Functional Medicine*, Institute for Functional Medicine, IFM Press.

Jones, D.S. (2010) *Textbook of Functional Medicine*, Institute for Functional Medicine, IFM Press.

LIFESTYLE AND MODERN FACTORS

Chrousos (2009) Stress and disorders of the stress system. *Nature Reviews Endocrinology*, 5(7), 374-381.

Hamilton & Ventura (2019) Birth rates for U.S. women continue to drop. NCHS Data Brief, No. 355.

CONVENTIONAL VS. FUNCTIONAL APPROACHES

Domar et al. (2018) The mind/body connection: the Boston IVF relaxation, stress management and mind/body program for infertile couples. *Applied Psychology*: Health and Well-Being, 10(3), 404-424.

Homan et al. (2007) The impact of lifestyle factors on reproductive performance in the general population and those undergoing infertility treatment. *Human Reproduction Update*, 13(3), 209-223.

SECTION II
MIND-BODY CONNECTION & FERTILITY

Boivin & Schmidt (2005) Infertility-related stress in men and women predicts treatment outcome 1 year later, *Fertility and Sterility*, 83(6), 1745-1752.

de Liz & Strauss (2005) A survey of reproductive experiences in women with polycystic ovary syndrome, *Health Care for Women International*, 26(1), 86-95.

Domar et al. (2000) Impact of group psychological interventions on pregnancy rates in infertile women, *Fertility and Sterility*, 73(4), 805-811.

GUT HORMONE CONNECTION

Baker et al. (2017) Estrogen-gut microbiome axis: Physiological and clinical implications, *Maturitas*, 103, 45-53.

Fuhrman et al. (2014) Associations of the fecal microbiome with urinary estrogens and estrogen metabolites in postmenopausal women, *Journal of Clinical Endocrinology & Metabolism*, 99(12), 4632-4640.

Kwa et al. (2016) The intestinal microbiome and estrogen receptor-positive female breast cancer, *Journal of the National Cancer Institute*, 108(8).

SYSTEMS BIOLOGY AND REPRODUCTIVE HEALTH

Chrousos et al. (1998) Interactions between the hypothalamic-pituitary-adrenal axis and the female reproductive system, *Annals of Internal Medicine*, 129(3), 229-240.

Makrigiannakis et al. (2011) Stress and reproduction: a tale of two systems, *Human Reproduction Update*, 17(4), 428-435.

INFLAMMATION AND FERTILITY

Ruder et al. (2014) Oxidative stress and antioxidants: exposure and impact on female fertility, *Human Reproduction Update*, 20(6), 873-886.

Agarwal et al. (2012) The effects of oxidative stress on female reproduction: a review, *Reproductive Biology and Endocrinology*, 10, 49.

SOCIAL SUPPORT AND REPRODUCTIVE OUTCOMES

Campagne (2013) Should fertilization treatment start with reducing stress? *Human Reproduction*, 28(11), 2955-2963.

Rooney & Domar (2018) The relationship between stress and infertility, *Dialogues in Clinical Neuroscience*, 20(1), 41-47.

ENVIRONMENTAL AND CULTURAL FACTORS

Gore et al. (2015) EDC-2: The Endocrine Society's second scientific statement on endocrine-disrupting chemicals, *Endocrine Reviews*, 36(6), E1-E150.

Woodruff et al. (2008) Environmental chemicals in pregnant women in the United States: NHANES 2003-2004, *Environmental Health Perspectives*, 119(6), 878-885.

INTEGRATIVE MEDICINE AND FERTILITY

Ernst & White (2001) Systematic review of systematic reviews of acupuncture published 1996-2000, *European Journal of Medicine*, 10(4-5), 227-235.

Zheng et al. (2012) Effects of acupuncture on pregnancy rates in women undergoing in vitro fertilization: a systematic review and meta-analysis, *Fertility and Sterility*, 97(3), 599-611.

FUNCTIONAL MEDICINE FOUNDATIONS

Bland (2014) *The Disease Delusion: Conquering the Causes of Chronic Illness for a Healthier, Longer, and Happier Life*. HarperWave.

Jones (2010) *Textbook of Functional Medicine*, Institute for Functional Medicine.

SECTION III
ENDOCRINE SYSTEM OVERVIEW

Chrousos et al. (1998) Interactions between the hypothalamic-pituitary-adrenal axis and the female reproductive system. *Annals of Internal Medicine*, 129(3), 229-240.

Herbison (2016) Control of puberty onset and fertility by gonadotropin-releasing hormone (GnRH) neurons, *Nature Reviews Endocrinology*, 12(8), 452-466.

ESTRADIOL

Hess (2003) Estrogen in the adult male reproductive tract: a review, *Reproductive Biology and Endocrinology*, 1, 52.

Nilsson et al. (2001) Mechanisms of estrogen action, *Physiological Reviews*, 81(4), 1535-1565.

PROGESTERONE

Graham & Clarke (1997) Physiological action of progesterone in target tissues, *Endocrine Reviews*, 18(4), 502-519.

Schindler et al. (2003) Classification and pharmacology of progestins, *Maturitas*, 46(Suppl 1), S7-S16.

ANDROGENS (TESTOSTERONE, DHEA, AND DHT)

Burger (2002) Androgen production in women, *Fertility and Sterility*, 77(Suppl 4), S3-S5.

Davison et al. (2005) Androgen levels in adult females: changes with age, menopause, and oophorectomy, *Journal of Clinical Endocrinology & Metabolism*, 90(7), 3847-3853.

CORTISOL AND PREGNENOLONE

Whirledge & Cidlowski (2010) Glucocorticoids, stress, and fertility, *Minerva Endocrinologica*, 35(2), 109-125.

Genazzani et al. (1998) Pregnenolone, progesterone and related derivatives in the brain, *Journal of Steroid Biochemistry and Molecular Biology*, 65(1-6), 293-299.

PROLACTIN

Freeman et al. (2000) Prolactin: structure, function, and regulation of secretion, *Physiological Reviews*, 80(4), 1523-1631.

Bole-Feysot et al. (1998) Prolactin (PRL) and its receptor: actions, signal transduction pathways and phenotypes observed in PRL receptor knockout mice, *Endocrine Reviews*, 19(3), 225-268.

THYROID HORMONES

Krassas et al. (2010) Thyroid function and human reproductive health, *Endocrine Reviews*, 31(5), 702-755.

Abalovich et al. (2007) Management of thyroid dysfunction during pregnancy and postpartum, *Journal of Clinical Endocrinology & Metabolism*, 92(8 Suppl), S1-S47.

HORMONE INTEGRATION AND FEEDBACK LOOPS

Plant (2015) Neuroendocrine control of the onset of puberty, *Frontiers in Neuroendocrinology*, 38, 73-88.

Meethal & Atwood (2005) The role of hypothalamic-pituitary-gonadal hormones in the normal structure and functioning of the brain, *Cellular and Molecular Life Sciences*, 62(3), 257-270.

HORMONE TESTING AND INTERPRETATION

Practice Committee of American Society for Reproductive Medicine (2015) - Diagnostic evaluation of the infertile female: a committee opinion, *Fertility and Sterility*, 103(6), e44-50.

Stricker et al. (2006) Establishment of detailed reference values for luteinizing hormone, follicle stimulating hormone, estradiol, and progesterone during different phases of the menstrual cycle, *Clinical Chemistry and Laboratory Medicine*, 44(7), 883-887.

SECTION IV
ENDOMETRIOSIS

Giudice, L.C. & Kao, L.C. (2004) Endometriosis, *Lancet*, 364(9447), 1789-1799.

Sampson, J.A. (1927) Peritoneal endometriosis due to the menstrual dissemination of endometrial tissue into the peritoneal cavity, *American Journal of Obstetrics and Gynecology*, 14(4), 422-469. (Classic reference)

Parazzini et al. (2013) Selected food intake and risk of endometriosis, *Human Reproduction*, 28(8), 1982-1989.

Halpern et al. (2015) The association between the combined oral contraceptive pill and insulin resistance, dysglycemia and dyslipidemia in women with polycystic ovary syndrome, *Journal of Reproductive Medicine*, 60(9-10), 377-382.

Missmer & Cramer (2003) The epidemiology of endometriosis, Obstetrics and Gynecology Clinics of North America, 30(1), 1-19.

CASTOR OIL

Vieira, C., et al. (2000). "Effect of ricinoleic acid in acute and subchronic experimental models of inflammation." *European Journal of Pharmacology*, 407(1-2), 109-116. doi: 10.1016/s0014-2999(00)00727-5

Grady, H. (1999). "Immunomodulation Through Castor Oil Packs." *Journal of Naturopathic Medicine*, 7(1).

Tunaru, S., et al. (2012). "Castor oil induces laxation and uterus contraction via ricinoleic acid activating prostaglandin EP3 receptors." *Proceedings of the National Academy of Sciences*, 109(23), 9179-9184. doi: 10.1073/pnas.1201627109

Rupa Health Case Study (2025). "A Functional Medicine Endometriosis Case Study: How Amber Recovered From Irregular Cycles and Heavy and Painful Periods."

PCOS

Rotterdam ESHRE/ASRM-Sponsored PCOS Consensus Workshop Group (2004) Revised 2003 consensus on diagnostic criteria and long-term health risks related to polycystic ovary syndrome, *Human Reproduction*, 19(1), 41-47.

Legro et al. (2013) Diagnosis and treatment of polycystic ovary syndrome: an Endocrine Society clinical practice guideline, *Journal of Clinical Endocrinology & Metabolism*, 98(12), 4565-4592.

Costello & Eden (2003) A systematic review of the reproductive system effects of inositol in women with polycystic ovary syndrome, *Archives of Gynecology and Obstetrics*, 268(4), 249-254.

Salehpour et al. (2012) A 12-week double-blind randomized clinical trial of vitamin D_3 supplementation on body fat mass in healthy overweight and obese women, *Nutrition Journal*, 11, 78.

Teede et al. (2018) Recommendations from the international evidence-based guideline for the assessment and management of polycystic ovary syndrome, *Human Reproduction*, 33(9), 1602-1618.

METFORMIN STUDIES

Legro et al. (2007) Clomiphene, metformin, or both for infertility in the polycystic ovary syndrome, *New England Journal of Medicine*. Found metformin restored ovulation in 78% of women with PCOS.

Tang et al. (2012) Insulin-sensitising drugs (metformin, rosiglitazone, pioglitazone, D-chiro-inositol) for women with polycystic ovary syndrome, oligo amenorrhoea and subfertility, Cochrane Database. Comprehensive review showing metformin improves ovulation rates.

Palomba et al. (2013) Metformin in women with PCOS pregnancy complications and pregnancy outcomes, *Human Reproduction Update*. Demonstrated reduced miscarriage rates with metformin continuation.

Tso et al. (2014) Metformin treatment before and during IVF or ICSI in women with polycystic ovary syndrome, Cochrane

Database. Showed improved clinical pregnancy rates with metformin in IVF cycles.

Glueck et al. (2008) Continuing metformin throughout pregnancy in women with polycystic ovary syndrome appears to safely reduce first-trimester spontaneous abortion, *Human Reproduction*.

Nestler, J.E., Jakubowicz, D.J., Evans, W.S., Pasquali, R. (1998). Effects of metformin on spontaneous and clomiphene-induced ovulation in the polycystic ovary syndrome. *New England Journal of Medicine*, 338(26), 1876-1880.

GLP-1 AGONIST STUDIES

Salamun et al. (2018) Liraglutide increases IVF pregnancy rates in obese PCOS women with poor response to first-line reproductive treatments, *European Journal of Endocrinology*.

Jensterle et al. (2019) Short-term effectiveness of low dose liraglutide in combination with metformin versus high dose liraglutide alone in treatment of obese PCOS, *European Journal of Endocrinology*.

Elkind-Hirsch et al. (2008) Comparison of single and combined treatment with exenatide and metformin on menstrual cyclicity in overweight women with polycystic ovary syndrome, *Journal of Clinical Endocrinology & Metabolism*.

Frøssing et al. (2018) Effect of liraglutide on anovulation in obese women with polycystic ovary syndrome: a randomized controlled trial, BMJ Open.

AMENORRHEA

Practice Committee of American Society for Reproductive Medicine (2008) Current evaluation of amenorrhea, *Fertility and Sterility*, 90(5 Suppl), S219-225.

Gordon et al. (2017) Functional hypothalamic amenorrhea: an Endocrine Society clinical practice guideline, *Journal of Clinical Endocrinology & Metabolism*, 102(5), 1413-1439.

Meczekalski et al. (2008) Functional hypothalamic amenorrhea and its influence on women's health, *Journal of Endocrinological Investigation*, 31(12), 1049-1056.

Loucks & Thuma (2003) Luteinizing hormone pulsatility is disrupted at a threshold of energy availability in regularly menstruating women, *Journal of Clinical Endocrinology & Metabolism*, 88(1), 297-311.

PREMATURE OVARIAN INSUFFICIENCY

European Society for Human Reproduction and Embryology (ESHRE) Guideline Group on POI et al. (2016) ESHRE Guideline: management of women with premature ovarian insufficiency, *Human Reproduction*, 31(5), 926-937.

Webber et al. (2016) ESHRE Guideline: management of women with premature ovarian insufficiency, *Human Reproduction*, 31(5), 926-937.

Coulam et al. (1986) Incidence of premature ovarian failure, *Obstetrics & Gynecology*, 67(4), 604-606.

PMS/PMDD

American College of Obstetricians and Gynecologists (2015) Committee Opinion No. 630: Screening for perinatal depression, *Obstetrics & Gynecology*, 125(5), 1268-1271.

Bertone-Johnson et al. (2005) Calcium and vitamin D intake and risk of incident premenstrual syndrome, *Archives of Internal Medicine*, 165(11), 1246-1252.

Freeman et al. (2010) Omega-3 fatty acids: evidence basis for treatment and future research in psychiatry, *Journal of Clinical Psychiatry*, 71(12), 1397-1409.

MALE FERTILITY

Agarwal et al. (2014) A unique view on male infertility around the globe, *Reproductive Biology and Endocrinology*, 12, 37.

Levine et al. (2017) Temporal trends in sperm count: a systematic review and meta-regression analysis, *Human Reproduction Update*, 23(6), 646-659.

Tremellen (2008) Oxidative stress and male infertility—a clinical perspective, *Human Reproduction Update*, 14(3), 243-258.

Safarinejad (2012) The effect of coenzyme Q_{10} supplementation on partner pregnancy rate in infertile men with idiopathic oligoasthenoteratozoospermia, *International Urology and Nephrology*, 44(3), 689-700.

EMF DANGER STUDIES

Agarwal et al. (2009) Effect of cell phone usage on semen analysis in men attending infertility clinic: an observational study, *Fertility and Sterility*. Found 25% reduction in sperm motility with cell phone use.

Fejes et al. (2005) Is there a relationship between cell phone use and semen quality?, *Archives of Andrology*, showed decreased sperm concentration and motility.

Avendaño et al. (2012) Use of laptop computers connected to internet through Wi-Fi decreases human sperm motility and increases sperm DNA fragmentation, *Fertility and Sterility*.

Adams et al. (2014) Effect of mobile telephones on sperm quality: A systematic review and meta-analysis, *Environment International*, comprehensive review showing consistent negative effects.

Liu et al. (2014) Association between mobile phone use and semen quality, *Andrology Journal*.

Zalata et al. (2015) In vitro effect of cell phone radiation on motility, DNA fragmentation and clusterin gene expression in human sperm, *International Journal of Fertility & Sterility*.

PERIMENOPAUSE/MENOPAUSE

Harlow et al. (2012) Executive summary of the Stages of Reproductive Aging Workshop + 10: addressing the unfinished agenda of staging reproductive aging, *Journal of Clinical Endocrinology & Metabolism*, 97(4), 1159-1168.

Practice Committee of the American Society for Reproductive Medicine (2014) Female age-related fertility decline, *Fertility and Sterility*, 101(3), 633-634.

INFECTIONS AND SCARRING

Ness et al. (2002) Effectiveness of inpatient and outpatient treatment strategies for women with pelvic inflammatory disease, *American Journal of Obstetrics and Gynecology*, 186(5), 929-937.

Wiesenfeld et al. (2012) Lower genital tract infection and endometritis: insight into subclinical pelvic inflammatory disease, *Obstetrics & Gynecology*, 120(2 Pt 1), 402-407.

Schenken (1989) *Pathogenesis in Endometriosis: Contemporary Concepts in Clinical Management*, Lippincott Williams & Wilkins.

Toth, A. (2004) *Fertile vs Infertile: How infections affect your fertility and your baby's health*. Fenestra Nooks Tuscon, Arizona.

Clear Passage: https://clearpassage.com

BLOOD-CLOTTING DISORDERS

Miyakis et al. (2006) International consensus statement on an update of the classification criteria for definite antiphospholipid syndrome, *Journal of Thrombosis and Haemostasis*, 4(2), 295-306.

Robertson et al. (2006) Thrombophilia in pregnancy: a systematic review, *British Journal of Haematology*, 132(2), 171-196.

Rai & Regan (2006) Recurrent miscarriage, *Lancet*, 368(9535), 601-611.

Klip et al. (2003) Epidemiological survey of the prevalence and fertility of women with Mayer-Rokitansky-Küster-Hauser syndrome in the Netherlands, *Human Reproduction*, 18(5), 909-912.

COMPREHENSIVE INFERTILITY

Practice Committee of American Society for Reproductive Medicine (2015) Diagnostic evaluation of the infertile female: a committee opinion, *Fertility and Sterility*, 103(6), e44-50.

Practice Committee of American Society for Reproductive Medicine (2015) Diagnostic evaluation of the infertile male: a committee opinion, *Fertility and Sterility*, 103(3), e18-25.

Zegers-Hochschild et al. (2017) The International Glossary on Infertility and Fertility Care, 2017, *Human Reproduction*, 32(9), 1786-1801.

SECTION V
STRESS REDUCTION AND FERTILITY

Domar et al. (2000) Impact of group psychological interventions on pregnancy rates in infertile women, *Fertility and Sterility*, 73(4), 805-811.

Rooney & Domar (2018) The relationship between stress and infertility, *Dialogues in Clinical Neuroscience*, 20(1), 41-47.

Louis et al. (2011) The effect of stress on women's fertility, *Journal of Women's Health*, 20(1), 41-48.

Campagne (2013) Should fertilization treatment start with reducing stress?, *Human Reproduction*, 28(11), 2955-2963.

POLYVAGAL THEORY AND THE NERVOUS SYSTEM

Porges, S.W. (2007) The polyvagal perspective, *Biological Psychology*, 74(2), 116-143.

Porges, S.W. (2009) The polyvagal theory: New insights into adaptive reactions of the autonomic nervous system, *Cleveland Clinic Journal of Medicine*, 76(Suppl 2), S86-S90.

Porges, S.W. (2011) *The Polyvagal Theory: Neurophysiological foundations of emotions, attachment, communication, and self-regulation*, W.W. Norton & Company.

Reed et al. (2018) Heart rate variability and fertility: a systematic review, *Psychoneuroendocrinology*, 95, 55-63.

Clancy et al. (2014) Non-invasive vagus nerve stimulation in healthy humans reduces sympathetic nerve activity, *Brain Stimulation*, 7(6), 871-877.

STRESS AND FERTILITY

Makrigiannakis et al. (2011) Stress and reproduction: a tale of two systems, *Human Reproduction Update*, 17(4), 428-435.

Campagne, D.M. (2013) Should fertilization treatment start with reducing stress? *Human Reproduction*, 28(11), 2955-2963.

Louis et al. (2011) The effect of stress on women's fertility, *Journal of Women's Health*, 20(1), 41-48.

VAGAL NERVE STIMULATION

Clancy et al. (2014) Non-invasive vagus nerve stimulation in healthy humans reduces sympathetic nerve activity, *Brain Stimulation*, 7(6), 871-877.

Huang et al. (2018) Effects of transcutaneous auricular vagus nerve stimulation on impaired glucose tolerance, *BMC Complementary and Alternative Medicine*, 18(1), 1-7.

HEART RATE VARIABILITY AND FERTILITY

Reed et al. (2018) Heart rate variability and fertility: a systematic review, *Psychoneuroendocrinology*, 95, 55-63.

Jarczok et al. (2013) Autonomic nervous system activity and workplace stressors, *Neuroscience & Biobehavioral Reviews*, 37(8), 1810-1823.

TRAUMA AND REPRODUCTIVE HEALTH:

Cwikel et al. (2004) Psychological interactions with infertility among women, *European Journal of Obstetrics & Gynecology and Reproductive Biology*, 117(2), 126-131.

Williams et al. (2013) Childhood trauma predicts antepartum mental health, *American Journal of Obstetrics and Gynecology*, 208(2), 127.e1-127.e7.

Kessler et al. (2012) The potential for heart rate variability biofeedback to improve health outcomes, *Applied Psychology: Health and Well-Being*, 4(2), 157-171.

Goessl et al. (2017) The effect of heart rate variability biofeedback training on stress and anxiety, *Psychological Medicine*, 47(15), 2578-2586.

MIND-BODY INTERVENTIONS

Domar et al. (2000) Impact of group psychological interventions on pregnancy rates in infertile women, *Fertility and Sterility*, 73(4), 805-811.

de Liz & Strauss (2005) A survey of reproductive experiences in women with polycystic ovary syndrome, *Health Care for Women International*, 26(1), 86-95.

NUTRITIONAL OPTIMIZATION

Chavarro et al. (2007) Use of multivitamins, intake of B vitamins, and risk of ovulatory infertility, *Fertility and Sterility*, 87(5), 1077-1085.

Gaskins et al. (2012) Diet and fertility: a review, *American Journal of Obstetrics and Gynecology*, 206(4), 327-333.

Vujkovic et al. (2010) Associations between dietary patterns and semen quality in men undergoing IVF/ICSI treatment, *Human Reproduction*, 25(6), 1372-1379.

SEED OILS AND INFLAMMATION

Attaman et al. (2012) Dietary fat and semen quality among men attending a fertility clinic, *Human Reproduction*, 27(5), 1466-1474.

Simopoulos (2008) The importance of the omega-6/omega-3 fatty acid ratio in cardiovascular disease and other chronic diseases, *Experimental Biology and Medicine*, 233(6), 674-688.

Patterson et al. (2012) Health implications of high dietary omega-6 polyunsaturated fatty acids, *Journal of Nutrition and Metabolism*, 2012, 539426.

Chiu, Y.H., Karmon, A.E., Gaskins, A.J., Arvizu, M., Williams, P.L., Souter, I., Rueda, B.R., Hauser, R., Chavarro, J.E. (2018) Serum omega-3 fatty acids and treatment outcomes among women undergoing assisted reproduction. *Human Reproduction*, 33(1), 156-165.

Alison Kane, RDN, LDN (2024) Seed Oils: Facts & Myths. Massachusetts General Hospital. October 16, 2024. Retrieved from www.massgeneral.org/news/article/seed-oils-facts-myths.

Chris Kresser, M. S. (2023) How industrial seed oils are making us sick. Retrieved from chriskresser.com/how-industrial-seed-oils-are-making-us-sick.

GUT HEALTH AND FERTILITY

Baker et al. (2017) Estrogen-gut microbiome axis: Physiological and clinical implications, *Maturitas*, 103, 45-53.

Kwa et al. (2016) The intestinal microbiome and estrogen receptor-positive female breast cancer, *Journal of the National Cancer Institute*, 108(8).

DETOXIFICATION AND ENVIRONMENTAL TOXINS

Gore et al. (2015) EDC-2: The Endocrine Society's second scientific statement on endocrine-disrupting chemicals, *Endocrine Reviews*, 36(6), E1-E150.

Woodruff et al. (2008) Environmental chemicals in pregnant women in the United States: NHANES 2003-2004, *Environmental Health Perspectives*, 119(6), 878-885.

Perkins et al. (2014) Serum BPA concentrations in pregnant women from a UK birth cohort: pregnancy and neonatal outcomes, *Environmental Research*, 129, 49-54.

HERBAL THERAPIES

Schellenberg (2001) Treatment for the premenstrual syndrome with agnus castus fruit extract: prospective, randomised, placebo controlled study, *BMJ*, 322(7279), 134-137.

Wuttke et al. (2003) Chaste tree (*Vitex agnus-castus*)—*pharmacology and clinical indications,* Phytomedicine, 10(4), 348-357.

Maheshwari et al. (2009) Multiple antioxidant, anticarcinogenic and immunomodulatory properties of Ashwagandha, *Biochemical Pharmacology*, 78(9), 1242-1251.

ACUPUNCTURE

Zheng et al. (2012) Effects of acupuncture on pregnancy rates in women undergoing in vitro fertilization: a systematic review and meta-analysis, *Fertility and Sterility*, 97(3), 599-611.

Jo & Lee (2017) Acupuncture for polycystic ovarian syndrome: a systematic review and meta-analysis, *Medicine*, 96(23), e7066.

SUPPLEMENT PROTOCOLS

Showell et al. (2013) Antioxidants for male subfertility, *Cochrane Database of Systematic Reviews*, (12), CD007411.

Bentov et al. (2014) The aging oocyte—can mitochondrial function be improved?, *Fertility and Sterility*, 101(1), 18-22.

Xu et al. (2018) Pretreatment with coenzyme Q10 improves ovarian response and embryo quality in low-prognosis young women with decreased ovarian reserve, *Reproductive Biology and Endocrinology*, 16(1), 29.

SPECIALIZED THERAPIES (HCG, PROGESTERONE, LDN)

Palomba et al. (2013) Metformin in women with PCOS pregnancy complications and pregnancy outcomes, *Human Reproduction Update*, 19(5), 477-496.

Palagiano et al. (2004) Low-dose naltrexone in the treatment of infertility in women with endometriosis, *Fertility and Sterility*, 82(6), 1540-1545.

Elsegood, L. (2018) *The LDN book: How a little-known generic drug—low dose naltrexone—could revolutionize treatment for autoimmune diseases, cancer, autism, depression, and more.* Chelsea Green Publishing.

INDEX

5-HTP, 158
abnormal bleeding patterns, 235
acne, 87, 121–23, 135, 154
acupuncture, 267, 311, 313–16, 318, 321, 341, 365, 380
adrenocorticotropic hormone (ACTH), 91, 108
age, 4, 10, 25, 28, 49, 51, 60, 82, 86, 114, 120, 134, 143, 145, 148, 151, 164–65, 170, 172, 187, 193, 213, 229–30, 240, 244–45, 247, 250, 286, 290, 328–29, 366, 374
aloe, 292
amenorrhea, 134–36, 138, 141–42, 261, 304, 322, 371–72
androgens, 21–22, 85, 87, 108, 121–22, 126, 226, 305, 314, 366
antibiotics, 11, 14, 189, 204, 208, 224, 341
antidepressants, 148, 166
anti-mullerian hormone (AMH), 1, 145, 151, 165, 226, 229, 288
antioxidants, 22, 117, 124, 168, 191, 217, 231, 242–43, 245, 248–49, 251, 280–83, 285–87, 289, 305, 334, 336, 341, 364, 380
anxiety, 4, 37, 41–43, 46, 56, 64, 84–85, 97, 154–56, 164, 268, 300, 326, 335, 378
arginine/L-Arginine, 191, 207, 234
ashwagandha, 124, 139, 158, 302, 304, 380

aspirin, 215, 218, 224
assisted reproductive technologies (ART), 189
astaxanthin, 282
B Complex, 128, 251, 330
berberine, 123, 159, 168, 205, 302, 330
betaine, 217, 292
biological, 29, 33–35, 39-40, 49, 52–53, 58-59, 61–62, 289, 321, 341–42, 376
birth control/oral contraceptive, 116, 122, 138, 148, 157, 160, 368
bloating, 35, 85, 153, 156, 348
blood, 7, 10, 14, 20–21, 28, 72, 77, 90–91, 106-7, 121–22, 136, 159–60, 171, 174, 177, 180, 199, 201, 203, 210, 212–20, 223–25, 230–31, 241, 256–57, 262, 277, 282, 298, 305, 308–9, 314, 323, 340–41, 350–51
blood thinners, 7, 14, 28, 224, 341
bone broth, 292
brain, 26, 36, 43, 70, 82, 86, 89–90, 92, 95, 136, 139, 154, 164, 180, 258, 274, 307–9, 311, 314, 366–67, 376–77

calcium, 117, 158–59, 169, 176, 300, 372
carnitine/L-carnitine, 150, 191, 231, 243
carotenoids, 274
cervix/cervical, 20–21, 72–73, 76, 78, 81–83, 99, 103–4, 174, 197–99, 203, 230, 234–35, 240, 303–4, 308, 311, 349
chiropractor, 309–310
chlamydia, 197
chlorella, 298
choline, 217
chromium, 123, 159, 168, 302
chronic infection, 204, 209
chrysin, 190
cinnamon, 159, 168, 301
clitoris, 73
Clomid (clomiphene), 122, 127, 138, 186, 189, 239, 369, 371
clotting, 28, 210–16, 218–21, 223–25, 340, 351
coconut oil, 274, 276, 278, 297
collagen, 205, 207, 281, 292
copper, 207, 302
CoQ10 (Ubiquinol), 149, 151, 168, 191–92, 231, 242–43, 245, 251, 280, 286, 320, 336
corticosteroids, 216

cortisol, 20, 22, 35, 37, 39, 41, 46, 56, 86, 89, 91–92, 107–8, 124, 158, 160, 190, 231, 243, 256, 258, 260, 284, 315, 334–35
culture, 51, 199, 204, 242
cysteine, 234, 281, 302
cytomegalovirus (CMV), 147
dandelion, 292
depression, 41, 154–55, 164, 261, 268, 372, 381
detoxification, 4, 6, 25, 35, 39, 77, 106, 117, 124, 149, 151, 169, 183, 192, 210–11, 220, 243, 278, 287, 290, 297–99, 320–21, 348, 395
difficulty conceiving, 165
difficulty concentrating, 144, 154
DIM (diindolylmethane), 158, 300
dopamine, 37, 40–41, 90, 93, 138
EGCG (green tea extract), 206
egg, 11, 21, 24–25, 28, 35-36, 39, 70–71, 76–77, 82–84, 96, 101–3, 106, 127, 148, 151–52, 167, 170–72, 174, 176, 186, 193–94, 202–3, 220, 222, 228–29, 231–32, 234, 241–42, 245, 249, 273, 275, 277–85, 287–91, 296, 305, 309, 334, 336–37
electromagnetic field (EMF), 11, 23, 27, 183–85, 187–88, 192, 285, 296, 298–99, 352, 373
embryo, 36, 71, 77, 84–85, 148, 193, 197–98, 203, 212, 223–24, 229–30, 242, 244–48, 272, 279, 286, 288–90, 316–17, 321, 326, 380
endometriosis, 12, 16, 27, 62, 78, 83, 113–19, 133, 147, 202, 300, 315, 325–27, 329, 340, 351, 358, 367–68, 374, 381
endometritis, 197, 199, 202, 208, 223–24
endometrium, 72, 82, 84, 142, 198, 203, 212
endorphin, 315, 325–28
EPA, 216, 282
epididymis, 75–76, 178–79
Epididymitis, 198
erectile dysfunction (ED), 179, 189, 305
estradiol, 81–83, 99, 103, 107–8, 136, 145, 165, 178, 226–27, 367
estriol, 82
estrogen, 20–21, 35–37, 40, 46, 70, 81, 83, 86–87, 93, 96, 99,

101, 103, 106–9, 117, 144–45, 148, 156, 158, 166, 169, 171, 190, 206, 233, 239, 300, 303–4, 363, 365, 379, 393
faith, 56, 60, 62, 245, 340–41, 344, 346
fallopian tubes, 70–71, 76–78, 113, 197–98, 201–3, 219, 226, 230, 240
fat, 37, 82, 92, 106, 274, 276–78, 280–82, 292, 303, 353, 369, 378
fatigue/tired, 46, 87, 91, 97, 145, 153, 305
fertility, 1, 4–7, 9–19, 21–29, 33–34, 37–53, 55–65, 69–70, 74, 77, 79, 81–85, 87, 90–94, 96–97, 99, 101–2, 106–7, 109, 113, 115, 118–21, 123, 126–30, 132–34, 139, 142, 148, 151–53, 155–57, 161–62, 165–67, 170, 172, 174, 176, 178–81, 183–88, 190, 193–95, 197–99, 202, 208–211, 219–22, 224–28, 233–36, 239, 242, 244, 246, 248–51, 255–63, 266–69, 271, 273–74, 276–77, 283, 288, 290–91, 295, 297, 300, 303–4, 306, 308–330, 333–38, 340–46, 348, 353, 355, 357–59, 361, 363–67, 371, 373–78, 380–81, 394–95

fetus, 72, 213
fimbriae, 71
fish oil, 115, 206, 216, 218, 224, 251, 275
folate/folic acid/methylfolate, 191, 211, 215, 217–18, 221, 224, 277, 282
follicle stimulating hormone (FSH), 1, 20, 22, 70, 101–3, 107–8, 136, 142, 145, 151–52, 165–66, 178, 185, 226–27, 229, 239, 367
gamma-aminobutyric acid (GABA), 37, 40, 90, 158
garlic, 205, 283, 292
genital tract infections, 374
ginger, 216, 277, 283, 301
glands/glandular tissue, 5, 26, 76, 79, 82, 84, 86, 90–92, 94, 96, 142, 180, 185
glucagon, 128
glucagon-like peptide-1 (GLP-1), 126, 128–33, 371
glutamine/L-Glutamine, 205, 292
glutathione, 124, 149, 168, 191, 217, 281, 290, 299
gonadotropins, 93, 189, 239, 322, 365
gonorrhea, 197

gut, 11, 22, 24–26, 28, 35, 39, 43, 106, 118–19, 124, 149, 190, 217, 228, 251, 291, 330, 334–35, 363, 379, 395
headache, 135, 153
heat, 97, 117–18, 178, 182–83, 187–88, 192, 230–31, 274, 276, 352
Heparin, 215
herpes, 197
history, 22–23, 114, 121, 125, 130, 135, 145, 155, 174, 178, 209, 213–15, 219, 223, 227, 262, 268, 314, 317, 329, 348, 351–52
holistic, 29, 34, 57, 62, 358
holy basil, 158
hope, 13, 27, 29, 60, 63–65, 290, 339, 343, 345–46
human chorionic gonadotropin (hCG), 6, 186, 189, 322, 325
human papillomavirus (HPV), 197
HVAC, 5, 94, 104, 319
hypothalamus, 36, 85, 96, 105, 142
ibuprofen, 116
implantation, 21–22, 28, 38, 72, 77, 81, 83–85, 91, 96, 99, 133, 156, 161, 171, 193, 197–99, 203, 210, 212–13, 219, 221–24, 244–45, 256, 260, 272, 275, 287, 290–91, 309, 314–15, 323–24, 326, 340
in vitro fertilization (IVF), 10, 14, 16, 50, 78, 127, 129, 148, 172, 189, 192, 200–201, 206, 213, 215, 222–23, 228, 241–49, 276, 283, 285, 287–89, 316–17, 321, 324, 327, 335–36, 341–42, 358, 362, 365, 369, 371, 378, 380
infection, 7, 36, 75, 147, 174, 177, 179–80, 189, 195, 197–99, 202, 204–5, 208–210, 222, 224–25, 231, 292, 341, 344, 374
infertility, 7, 9–10, 14, 16, 28, 36, 42, 62, 87, 94, 114, 133, 142, 189, 195, 202, 213, 219, 227, 240, 244–45, 250, 305, 316, 321, 325, 329, 334, 361, 363–64, 369, 373, 376–78, 381
inflammation, 6, 13–14, 25, 28, 35-36, 39, 63, 77, 90, 106, 113, 116, 118, 127–28, 133, 159, 168, 177, 180, 197–99, 205, 209, 212, 214, 217, 223–25, 244, 272, 275–78, 283, 291, 296, 309, 315, 325–27, 334–35, 340–42, 368
inhibin, 145, 165

inositol/D-chiro-inositol, 123, 159, 251, 302, 330, 369
insomnia, 97, 148, 166
insulin, 20, 37, 40, 91–92, 96, 105–6, 120, 122–23, 125–33, 159, 168, 227, 246, 277, 301, 326, 368–69
intracytoplasmic sperm injection (ICSI), 189, 192, 242, 370, 378
intrauterine insemination, 7, 189, 198, 240
intrauterine insemination (IUI), 7, 16, 189, 198, 239–40, 316, 324, 341
iodine, 96, 140, 150, 302
iron, 302, 330
irregular periods, 151
irritability, 144, 154, 164
labia, 73
letrozole (Femara), 122, 138, 239
licorice, 303
liver, 25, 90, 96, 117, 124, 149, 158, 169, 192, 243, 257, 278, 305, 323, 348
Lovenox (enoxaparin), 215, 218, 223–24
low dose naltrexone (LDN), 216, 325–28, 379, 381
luteinizing hormone (LH), 20, 22, 70, 82, 101–3, 107–8, 136, 142, 178, 185, 226–27, 233, 239, 322, 367, 372
lycopene, 191
maca, 304
magnesium, 96, 115, 117, 139, 150, 158–60, 168, 190, 217, 251, 290, 301, 330, 335
male, 9, 62, 74, 76, 85–87, 96, 121, 174, 176, 178–81, 184–85, 188–90, 193–95, 198, 206, 226–27, 240, 244, 267, 304, 316–17, 322, 326, 329, 350, 352, 362, 365, 373, 375, 380
manganese, 207
marshmallow root, 292
melatonin, 51, 53, 168, 231, 282, 284
menstrual cycle, 82, 84, 96, 121–22, 134, 144, 151, 155, 165, 168, 303, 349, 367
Metformin, 122, 126–28, 130–33, 369-370, 380
migraine, 36, 153, 213
milk thistle, 124, 149, 169, 191, 292
miscarriage, 1, 10, 28, 38, 85, 97, 127, 156, 161, 183, 193,

221, 223, 272, 289, 324, 335, 369, 375
mold, 147, 195, 295–97, 393
MSM, 299
multivitamin, 378
muscle pain, 153
mycoplasma, 197, 199
myometrium, 72
N-acetylcysteine (NAC), 149, 151, 168, 191, 205, 231, 234, 243, 251, 281, 299, 302, 330
nervous system, 27, 41, 46, 56, 84, 117, 140, 158, 256–69, 307–313, 315, 335, 376–77
night sweats, 135, 144, 164–65
NSAIDs, 116, 156, 292
nutraceutical products, 250
nutrition, 23–24, 28, 51, 77–78, 115, 117, 126, 129–30, 136, 139–40, 149, 159–60, 168–69, 218, 230–31, 233, 248, 271, 276, 278, 280, 287, 300, 320, 328, 344, 353, 369, 379
omega-3 (Fish Oil), 115, 117, 124, 139, 149, 159, 168, 190, 206, 216, 218, 224, 242–43, 251, 275–76, 278, 282, 320, 336, 373, 378–79
omega-6, 190, 272, 274–76, 378–79
oregano oil, 205
ovaries/ovary, 12, 70–71, 76–77, 82, 86, 105, 113, 120–22, 127, 133, 137, 139, 142–43, 146, 165, 202, 226, 257, 299, 308–9, 314, 363, 368–71, 378
ovulation, 20–21, 38, 70–71, 76, 82, 84–85, 92–93, 96, 99–100, 102–4, 108, 115, 117, 120–22, 126–27, 129–30, 132–33, 138, 141–42, 148, 151, 153, 156–57, 165–66, 170, 174, 226, 232–34, 239–40, 256, 260, 277, 279–80, 288–89, 314–15, 322–24, 369, 371
oxytocin, 41, 45, 48, 56
pain, 37, 113–17, 129, 156, 180, 200–201, 204, 209, 246, 262, 308, 310, 326, 349, 351–52
painful intercourse, 144
PCOS, 12, 16, 21, 37, 62, 87, 105, 120–23, 125–27, 129–30, 133–34, 301, 314, 326, 351, 368–69, 371, 381
pelvic inflammatory disease (PID), 202, 351, 374
Phosphatidylserine, 158
pituitary, 21, 41, 56, 91–92, 94, 96, 105, 136–37, 139, 142, 157, 185–86, 303, 314

Polyvagal theory, 259–60, 263
power, 57, 60, 81, 83, 120, 122, 124, 126, 133, 246, 249, 334, 345
PQQ, 149, 168, 191, 231, 243, 281
prayer, 58, 60, 62–63, 65, 341
prebiotic, 118, 124, 190, 205, 292
pregnenolone, 89, 91, 105, 167, 366
premenstrual dysphoric disorder (PMDD), 153–56, 161–62, 372
premenstrual syndrome (PMS), 12, 35, 85, 101, 103–4, 144, 153–56, 159–62, 164, 288, 300, 303, 335, 349, 372, 380
prenatal vitamins, 221
probiotics, 118, 158, 190
progesterone, 6, 20, 22, 36, 38–39, 41, 46, 70, 83–85, 93, 96, 99, 101, 103–4, 107–9, 115, 125, 142, 148, 155–58, 160–61, 165, 167, 171, 224, 226, 288, 300–301, 303, 323–25, 335, 337, 366–67
prolactin, 92–94, 107, 122, 136–38, 146, 178, 226–27, 303, 366
prostate, 87, 174, 178, 198
quercetin, 205
Rehmannia, 150
resveratrol, 150, 168, 231, 243, 282
reverse T3, 22, 95
rosemary extract, 300
safe, 131, 142, 186, 256, 258–60, 263, 267, 269
saliva, 107
Schisandra, 305
scrotum, 74, 182
seed oils, 271–77, 283, 379
selenium, 96, 140, 150, 191–92, 231, 302, 336
seminal vesicles, 198
serotonin, 36, 40–41, 156, 158
sexually transmitted disease (STD), 174
sexually transmitted infection (STI), 197, 199, 209, 351–52
Shatavari, 303
social, 29, 33, 42, 45–49, 51, 60–61, 103, 154, 233, 259–61, 263, 267
sodium, 298
sperm, 9, 11, 20, 24–25, 35–36, 39, 71, 73–78, 81–82, 87, 96, 107, 174, 176–89, 191, 193–94, 197–99, 203, 206, 219–20, 222,

224, 226–27, 229, 231–32, 234, 240–42, 249, 267, 271–73, 275–79, 296, 304–5, 316–17, 321–22, 326, 334, 336, 350, 361, 373–74
spiritual, 29, 33, 53, 55–61, 245
spironolactone, 122
SSRIs, 156
supplements, 6, 24–25, 28, 77, 104, 115, 117, 123–25, 130–32, 139, 149, 158, 168, 190, 205, 233, 243, 269, 280, 286–89, 300–302, 320, 341, 344, 353, 355
surgery, 7, 14, 16, 115–16, 138, 145, 147, 178, 200–202, 208, 223–24, 341, 351–52, 358
swelling, 153, 180, 352
T3 (Free T3), 22, 38, 94–97, 226, 302
T4 (Free T4), 22, 94–97, 226, 302
testes/testis, 74, 76–77, 86, 105, 178, 180, 299
testosterone, 20, 39, 41, 46, 70, 74, 85–87, 101–3, 120, 122, 136, 167, 171, 178, 182, 185–87, 189–91, 226–27, 256, 267, 304–5, 322, 350
theanine, 158, 251

thyroid, 11, 20–22, 35, 37–38, 41, 46, 91, 93–97, 105, 107, 122, 136–37, 145–46, 148, 150–51, 155, 166, 190, 226–27, 302, 326, 350, 366–67
thyroid stimulating hormone (TSH), 38, 96–97, 226
TMG, 217
toxins, 6, 13–14, 22, 77, 119, 124, 145, 147, 149, 169, 181–82, 187, 191–92, 195, 220, 227, 230–31, 244, 295, 299, 310, 320–21, 336–38, 344, 348
trauma, 42, 202, 261–63, 267–68, 352, 377
Tribulus, 304
tryptophan, 158
turmeric/curcumin, 115, 159, 168, 207, 216, 251, 277, 283, 300–301
tyrosine, 96, 302
ureaplasma, 197, 199
urethra/urethral, 75, 174
urinary tract infection, 174
urine, 108, 174, 298
uterus/uterine, 7, 20–21, 70–73, 76–78, 81, 83–84, 92, 99, 101, 113, 118–19, 121, 133, 137–38, 146, 161, 171, 197, 199, 201–4, 206, 212, 216, 222–24,

226, 230, 240, 242, 244, 246, 257, 260, 305–6, 308–9, 314, 340, 368
vaccination, 145, 147, 180
vagina/vaginal, 36, 72–73, 75–76, 135, 137, 144, 148, 164, 166, 174, 197, 199, 205, 208, 323
vagus nerve, 264–65, 376–77
viral infection, 145, 180
vitamin B, 139, 157–58, 301
vitamin B12 (methylcobalamin), 217–18, 224
vitamin B2 (riboflavin), 217
vitamin C, 124, 149, 168, 191, 207, 217, 281, 290–91, 301, 336
vitamin D, 38, 140, 149, 155, 159, 190, 215, 217–18, 242, 245, 251, 274, 282, 369, 372
vitamin D3, 251, 282
vitamin E (tocopherol), 117, 150, 168, 191, 217, 231, 274, 281, 336
vitex/chasteberry, 157, 160, 301, 303, 380
vulva, 73
zinc, 96, 139, 150, 159, 168, 174, 176, 190–92, 205, 231, 251, 290, 292, 300, 302, 330, 336

ABOUT THE AUTHOR

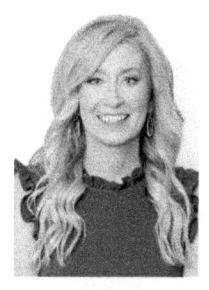

Stephanie Gray, DNP, MS, ARNP, AGNP-C, ABAAHP, FAARFM, is a functional medicine provider who helps men and women build sustainable and optimal health and longevity so that they can focus on what matters most to them!

She has been working as a nurse practitioner since 2009. Dr. Gray completed her doctorate, focusing on estrogen metabolism, from the University of Iowa in 2011. Additionally, she has a Master's in Metabolic Nutritional Medicine from the University of South Florida's Medical School. Her expertise lies within integrative, anti-aging, and functional medicine.

Dr. Gray is arguably one of the Midwest's most credentialed female healthcare providers, combining many certifications and trainings. In 2013 she completed an Advanced fellowship in Anti-Aging Regenerative and Functional Medicine and became the first BioTe certified provider in Iowa to administer hormone pellets. She is one of Dr. Nirala Jacobi's SIBO doctor-approved practitioners and is also one of Dr. Jill Crista's certified mold-literate providers. She has appeared on numerous podcasts, summits, and TV interviews and is a contributor to various health publications. She is the initial author of the FNP Mastery App and an Amazon best-selling author of her first book *Your Longevity Blueprint*.

Dr. Gray is the host of the Your Longevity Blueprint podcast and co-founder of Your Longevity Blueprint Nutraceuticals with her husband, Eric. After her own ten-year fertility journey, she now also specializes in helping couples optimize their reproductive health through functional medicine approaches. They enjoy spending time outdoors with their sons, William and Michael. They founded the Integrative Health and Hormone Clinic in Hiawatha, Iowa.

If *Your Fertility Blueprint* helped you understand how your body's systems work together, you've already begun the foundational work of longevity. Now it's time to complete your health renovation.

In *Your Longevity Blueprint*, I show you how the same functional medicine principles that optimized your fertility can transform your entire health span. The gut healing, detoxification, and hormone balancing you've learned aren't just for conception—they're the foundation for thriving throughout your life.

Inside *Your Longevity Blueprint*, you'll discover how to:

- Restore gut health
- Keep your spine in line
- Influence your genetics
- Replete nutritional deficiencies
- Detoxify your body
- Optimize your hormones
- Reduce Cardiovascular disease
- Strengthen your immune system

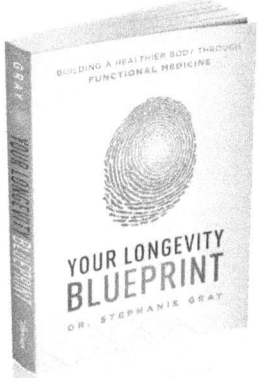

Your body is your home, and your functional medicine provider acts as your contractor and builder—giving your body the foundation, framework, and electricity it needs. Where conventional medicine treats symptoms, functional medicine discovers the root cause through your unique health "fingerprint."

IMAGINE WHAT LIFE WOULD BE LIKE WITH TRUE LONG TERM HEALTH. LET'S LIVE LONG TOGETHER! WELLNESS IS WAITING.

Available now wherever books are sold.

www.ingramcontent.com/pod-product-compliance
Lightning Source LLC
Chambersburg PA
CBHW020453030426
42337CB00011B/90